"Saida is a truly inspirational instructor and writer who lives what she teaches. You can't help but feel your own sense of joy and self-love expand in her presence. She has an extraordinary ability to assist other women in finding their own passion and spiritual paths. She is a gift to us all."

— RACHEL CARLTON ABRAMS MD
AUTHOR OF *The Multi-Orgasmic Woman*

"This is the book we've all been waiting for! Saida has interpreted The Tao from male dominated teachings into the warmth and beauty of feminine perspective. There is enough material here to transform the mundane into the sacred."

— CAROLINE MUIR
CO-AUTHOR OF *Tantra: The Art of Conscious Loving*
AND FOUNDER OF THE DIVINE FEMININE INSTITUTE

"Saida Désilet's new book, Emergence of the Sensual Woman, *is a treasure for any woman seeking to enhance her knowledge, awareness and skills regarding her own sensual, erotic and orgasmic capacities. This book opens up our understanding of sensuality, sexuality and orgasm in a clear, sensitive and fresh way while revealing the specific Taoist practices which enhance our feminine musculature, orgasmic response mechanisms, psychic energy, and feeling pathways. Truly, this book will be a handbook and guide for women for generations to come."*

— PATRICIA TAYLOR
AUTHOR OF *Expanded Orgasm*

Emergence
of the
Sensual Woman

Emergence of the Sensual Woman

Awakening Our Erotic Innocence

Saida Désilets

Jade Goddess Publishing

Wailea, Maui

Disclaimer

The information presented in this book is based on the author's personal experience as a Universal Tao Instructor. It is for the purpose of education and for the empowerment of each woman to reclaim her divine birthright: succulent bliss. The techniques explained are to be used with discretion and reader's liability. The author is not responsible or liable in any manner for any body sensations, experiences and possible issues resulting from applying the techniques contained in this book. Success in these practices is directly related to the amount of time dedicated to them.

For every woman willing to remember who she truly is: the living, breathing expression of the Divine Feminine whose essence is Succulent Love.

For every man willing to embrace his own feminine essence and honor the same in all the women in his life.

CONTENTS

It is with joy in my heart that I write this foreword for Saida's *Emergence of the Sensual Woman*. Saida intrigues me with her innovative style of instructing the female sexual practice and her embodiment of a very good quality of yin energy. Her Jade Goddess teachings blend not only the powerful practices from the Universal Healing Tao system, it also brings in a version of the female sexual practice that I have known was missing from the regular Taoist teachings. After extending an invitation for Saida to share her teachings at my Tao Garden Center in Thailand, I also asked her to work intimately with Dr. Rachel Abrams and me as a resource for our book, *The Multi-Orgasmic Woman*.

I believe *Emergence of the Sensual Woman* will be a unique and important contribution to both the Taoist community and mainstream readers. This book fuses both philosophical and technical concepts in an easy, thought-provoking manner, inspiring readers to understand the Taoist way as a practical, life-enhancing path.

The Tao way is the balanced way and, as humanity now moves to bring into balance the yin/feminine chi, this book shall be an essential resource for facilitating this global shift. As more women understand their power and live in harmony with their yin and yang chi, more balance and harmony will be felt within the population as a whole. This book reveals a wealth of techniques expertly shared not only in the words, but equally in Saida's presence. She lives these teachings. A teacher who embodies the powerful qualities of yin is a gift, and it is an honor to have her as a representative of the Universal Tao system.

MANTAK CHIA
Founder of the Universal Tao and Healing Tao System
June 2006

Before investigating a new way of perceiving sexuality and sensuality, it may be helpful to understand a little more about me and how I came to write *Emergence of the Sensual Woman*. In 1999, I was introduced to the Taoist teachings. Within a month of diligent practice, the results were so substantial that my dedication and exploration of qi gong (energy practice) and sexual energy became fully ignited. These results are woven into the chapters of this book as they were integral to my creation of the Art of Succulent Living and Jade Goddess teachings—a deep exploration of the full potential of being a completely activated and vibrantly succulent woman in the 21st century.

I did not wish to write just another sex or self-help book for women, but rather to extend an invitation to the reader to move into herself, into the very essence of the Feminine. Acknowledging that our DNA, the galaxies, and everything we call energy moves in a spiral, I chose my vision and words to reflect this harmonious and natural non-linear pattern. As women, we are guides of this spiral path, weaving our emotions, intuitions, intellect, sexuality and spirit into all that we create, every day of our lives. Falling out of this rhythm results in disease (be it mental, emotional, physical, or spiritual); thus, investing in our return to a natural sense of integration and free-flowing sensuality can only be for our greatest health and wealth.

This book is an invitation to each and every woman to ignite her own inner wisdom, radiant passion, and erotic innocence. It is a work of love dedicated to the light-hearted, fun, juicy, sacred aspects of sexual energy and its cultivation. Whether this is your first time looking into these teachings or whether you have already established a well-worn path, may this book act as a support tool for your unique journey of self-discovery and self-cultivation.

Chapters one through six cover the Art of Succulent Living, a set of concepts and beliefs used to expand our understanding of the world in which we live. Chapters seven through twelve cover the technical practices of the Jade Goddess teachings. If this is your first exposure to these teachings, it would be valuable to read these chapters a few times prior to doing the practices. If you are an advanced practitioner, these chapters will serve as a review and assist you in deepening your embodiment of these teachings. I also welcome male readers to enter the secret world of the Feminine as guests, and I encourage them to view the content with the understanding that it was written specifically as a woman's guide to cultivating her succulence.

"May the Divine Feminine awaken within you and may your path be blessed with an abundance of succulence. Live life fully."

ACKNOWLEDGMENTS

I would like to extend my deepest gratitude to the many who encouraged me to write this book and who supported me during the entire creative process, either through providing material as stories and quotes or for facilitating the actual production of this manuscript. More specifically, I would like to mention the generous contributions of the following people: Dr. Rachel Abrams, my friend and inspiration; Charlie Cantrell, the man who opened the door; Master Mantak Chia, my most respected teacher; Dr. Joan Heartfield, my friend and Ph.D supervisor; Shalene Takara, my editor and book designer; as well as my community of colleagues for verification and insight.

I would also like to thank all the professionals in the qi gong, tantra, and sexology field for their wisdom and contributions, especially Rebecca Chalker, Dr. Stephan T. Chang, Dr. Winnifred Cutler, Nik Douglas and Penny Slinger, Lonny S. Jarrett, Alice Kahn Ladis, Dr. Newman Kunti Lin, Caroline Muir, John Perry, Dr. Gary Shubach, Beverly Whipple, and Michael Winn. In addition, I would like to acknowledge my parents, all my teachers, my sister, and my beloved friends for believing in me and cheering me on.

I am delighted that you have chosen to embark on this journey with me. Together we will explore the vast and powerful mysteries of our feminine essence. It takes courage to redefine ourselves beyond the constructs of our current understanding of what it means to be a woman. This path is one of compassion, acceptance and growth. It is a tender moment when we step into ourselves and awaken our erotic innocence. Let's savor this experience by allowing it to unfold through letting go of our expectations and opening ourselves to limitless possibilities. Now let's look at what lies ahead on our path to emerging as sensual women.

THE ART OF SUCCULENT LIVING

When we choose to awaken our true nature as women, we realize that we are in truth very much alive and connected to all of life. This realization as well as the ability to surrender to our innate beauty as feminine expressions of the Divine is part of living a succulent life. To live succulently means allowing our life force to flow freely through us, making us supple, vibrant, inspired, inspiring, and ecstatically alive.

EXPLORING A NEW VIEW OF SEXUALITY AND SENSUALITY

Whether we are venturing into this world for the first time, or we have already carved a path in the realm of sacred sexuality, this book invites us into our feminine essence. Embracing our sexual/sensual nature, opening our heart, radiating out love without fear, and choosing to be a conscious creator of our life is the Art of Succulent Living in action.

SUCCULENT AUTHENTICITY

Some aspects of this book will feel like they have always been a part of what we know and while others may feel foreign. I have made a special effort to include and share intimate stories in a candid way to invite a space of deep authenticity and truth—a space where true healing and learning can occur. When we create a space of openness, acceptance, genuine trust, and curiosity without making anything right or wrong, good or bad, we invite ourselves to experience new levels of self-understanding, self-love, and self-acceptance.

FLOWING WITH SUCCULENT CHANGES

"What happens when I do all these things, and I change in ways I am not familiar with and attempt to live in the real world?" This is a common question often left unanswered by most of the schools that teach the sacred teachings of sexual energy cultivation. Therefore, I have dedicated the first half of the book to addressing this phenomenon, incorporating both accounts from my personal experience and the observations of thousands of people in workshops and seminars worldwide.

Practical Path to Succulent Living

The Art of Succulent Living isn't just theory or philosophy. It also contains practices designed to cultivate aliveness in every part of our being. These practices, that I call the Jade Goddess teachings, are a combination of practices that have been passed down through thousands of years as well as my own innovative techniques. While some practices appear nonsexual-sensual or simplistic in nature, the foundation practices lead to revitalizing and balancing the entire person (body-mind-spirit). Once a strong, clear base is formed, we are free to expand our sexual/sensual experience to its limitless possibilities.

Re-Union of the Feminine and Masculine

Alive sexuality and sensuality move us from an era when women were suppressed, controlled or diminished in some way, to a new era where men and women live together in exalted harmony. This new time embraces the gift of allowing the Masculine and Feminine energies to exist in harmony both inwardly and outwardly. When our inner and outer realities become more tangibly one, our yin and yang harmoniously function and express themselves throughout our existence.

Emergence of the Sensual Woman

Let's now begin this magnificent journey into ourselves, into the understanding of who we really are through thought-provoking concepts and easy, fun, practical, and transformative techniques. At this point, I want to remind each woman that she already knows all of this and to fully trust her own inner wisdom and guidance above anything written herein. I am simply a guide along the way.

With deepest respect,

Saida

Saida Désilets
Maui, Hawaii, July 2006

Sex is not a technique, a certain orgasm or partner, sex is our innate inner vitality. Sex chi/energy creates new life in the form of babies and the same chi/energy also creates vitality and radiance within us.

It is important to remember that we are born with this energy. It is our birthright. It is within each and every one of us to fully enjoy and cultivate this ecstatic chi/energy.

Without sex chi, life could not continue. However, misuse or misunderstanding of sex chi prevents us from fully experiencing the immense power of creation that sits dormant in our pelvis.

It is a total privilege to share my version of sexual energy cultivation. With the intention of honoring the wisdom and guidance within each woman, I now present the Emergence of the Sensual Woman.

PART ONE

The Art of
Succulent Living
Philosophy

CHAPTER ONE

The Art of Succulent Living

The Essence of the Sacred Teachings
of the Jade Goddess

The return home isn't always easy
life tests our truth
our fortitude, our stamina
our core beliefs

when in a difficult stretch
when the horizon is hidden
around that next bend
take heed of this:
It is only a test to see if you remember, do you?

Do you know why you are here?
Those things that you call challenges
are really magnificent gifts
bestowed with love and a sprinkle of humor

If we can remember together
that laughter and love
are the main ingredients
we will stop pretending
that we have to be serious
Recognizing that our freedom
true freedom
lies in our own understanding of our why

So why are you here?

WE LIVE IN A WORLD THAT IS BARREN OF SUCCULENCE, a modern world designed to suck us dry. As youth, we begin our lives plump and vital. Yet just a few years later, many of us have grown into weary, drained, joyless adults. Up until this moment, we have had two choices for defining our feminine **essence**: being considered a slut or frigid. Between these two extremes, however, exists the succulent world of the sensual woman. This world is rich with vibrant, confident, sexually open, magnetic, conscious, and radiant women. In this world, the Feminine has the power to enchant and to heal.

How often do we encounter a succulent, sensual woman? Up until now not very often, simply because it has not been *safe* for us to express our succulence and sensuality. The world we currently live in greets the feminine essence with bitterness, hostility and violence. It is scary to be juicy. To become our sensual selves and embrace our fullness as women, we must realize that who we are will create reverberations in this dry world. How can we not? When rains fall on a barren dessert, the excitement of freshness and new life stirs the dust from the ground and creates a commotion. Similarly, as sensual women entering a space that is barren of life, we excite a reaction. Whether the reaction is positive or negative depends on the environment we are in. As sensual women, we recognize these reactions as natural and through our grace, ease, and joy, we embrace all responses to our aliveness.

The Art of Succulent Living

The Art of Succulent Living is having the awareness and the capacity to live life in such a way that each moment serves to bring greater joy, ease, and vitality to us as women. It is what brings about our true emergence as sensual women. The art of living a succulent life is our choice to create moment-to-moment opportunities that lead to a sense of greater peace, radiance and personal empowerment. It is the ability to choose love, to choose life, and to choose freedom regardless of current conditions. Maintaining an attitude that makes our life as delightful and aware as possible is just one aspect of this art, and just like any art, succulent living incorporates a set of practices and philosophies that aid us in accessing our own innate creativity and unique expression. The philosophies and practices in this book are designed to give us an understanding of our innate feminine essence and provide the skills necessary to develop our own art, to be the master of our own true sensual selves, and to allow our sensual selves to emerge. Thus, living as sensual women is an act of renewing our faith and trust in ourselves while cultivating those aspects of our bodies, minds, and spirits which are **life-giving**.

As sensual women practicing this art, we see each and every moment as an opportunity, rich with beauty, vitality, and the possibility to embrace what is.

Accessing Succulence Through Sensuality

Sensuality is how we perceive the world through our sense of taste, touch, sight, sound, and smell. The more sensual we are, the more enjoyment we are able to derive from the things we are sensing. Succulence arises from our sexual energy and vitality. In order to become more succulent we must become more sensually aware through our heightened senses. Emerging as sensual women naturally occurs as a result of practicing the Art of Succulent Living. This involves accessing and refining our senses, increasing our capacity to experience pleasure, and in turn, awakening our sexuality through transforming these sensations into vitality and succulence.

Many of us walk through life merely experiencing "the same-old, same-old". This is because our senses are underdeveloped and we see life through the lens of "life is bland, boring, or mundane". On the other hand, as sensual women with awakened sensual selves (or essences), we perceive the world through a lens of heightened and developed sensuality. It is this part that allows us to experience the fullness and abundance of our own sensuality and to live succulent lives.

The Different Aspects of the Art of Succulent Living

Every art is multi-faceted. To master an art, well-rounded training in all its facets is essential. For example, training as a dancer requires knowledge not only of dance techniques, but also anatomy, nutrition, music, dance history and cultivation of one's own unique creative expression. Similarly, the harmonious blending of the Art of Succulent Living principles with the practices of the Jade Goddess teachings encompass an array of concepts which include:

- ❖ living in the world as sensual women
- ❖ understanding and managing our power with integrity
- ❖ living with more conscious awareness
- ❖ creating more effective and meaningful interactions with our communities.

Discovering a wealth of physical practices based on the Jade Goddess teachings which include:

- ❖ the potential of Omni-Orgasm
- ❖ dynamics of the Divine Masculine and Divine Feminine energies

- ❖ sexual qi gong for changing one's sexual/sensual physiology
- ❖ sexual anatomy
- ❖ sexual reflexology
- ❖ the phenomenon of female ejaculation (ambrosia)

Without a thorough understanding of how the cultivation of sexual energy works within our modern-day reality, its practical value would be next to nothing. This is why the Jade Goddess approach is two-fold, balancing the physical practice with grounded philosophy.

How did the Jade Goddess and the Art of Succulent Living Teachings begin?

Before we begin tending to the gentle emergence of our sensual selves, it is helpful for us to first understand how these teachings originated and what their modern-day applications are. That said, let's briefly take a look at the history of this lineage before we embark.

Ancient **Taoists** were both scientists and artists who explored the vast potential of the body and all its energetic attributes. After thousands of years investigating human nature, they discovered that the key to a long, healthy life resided in the cultivation of their sexual essence. This led them to create the Taoist way or what we currently know as **Taoist sexual qi gong**. As a modern Taoist, Mantak Chia explains, "Ancient Taoist sages believed we were born to be immortal. We become mortal by draining ourselves of chi through engaging in excessive sexual activity, indulging in negative emotions, and depending only on material sources to supply our life force." These ancient Taoists teachings, however, were not available to the general public as they were considered to be very potent and powerful—too powerful for the average person. Thus, sexual qi gong remained a well-kept secret, reserved solely for royalty and the lineage holders that inherited the tradition.

In the 1970s, something occurred which had not happened before. Master Yi Eng authorized his student, Mantak Chia, to bring these teachings to the West. Master Chia agreed and continued to investigate and develop the Taoist practices through his understanding of Chinese medicine and the use of Western scientific research. In 1979, he brought these teachings to the United States and created the Universal Tao System, a blend of ancient Taoist wisdom and modern medical research, giving us all access to this ancient wisdom.

With both increased sales in female sexual qi gong literature and in the attendance in female sexual qi gong seminars, it has become evident that this sexual practice is rising in popularity as more and more women are drawn to exploring their sexuality through this respected and natural system of the Universal Tao. Mantak Chia, a Taoist master, along with Dr. Rachel Abrams, a Western medical doctor, produced a valuable book: *The Multi-Orgasmic Woman*. Together they interwove the Taoist wisdom with current Western medical research to produce a thorough resource for women desiring to explore the women's Taoist practice of sexual energy cultivation. They found that women who work with the **Jade Egg** (an egg-shaped piece of Jade used for exercising and harmonizing the female sexual organs) and the other practices found in this book could lessen or eliminate **PMS** and menopausal symptoms, aid in fertility and cancer prevention (of the breasts and genitals), and stimulate a much wider range of orgasmic experiences. According to Dr. Abrams, "In my personal and professional experience, Taoist sexual practices are the most powerful techniques for sexual healing and transformation that I have encountered. "

Keeping in harmony with Chia's and Abram's work, this book not only uses the ancient wisdom of the Taoist sexual qi gong practices, but it also contributes to the lineage by deepening and expanding the Jade Egg practice.

The Jade Goddess is the name of the women's sexual teachings I developed using the Jade Egg. The Art of Succulent Living philosophy accompanies these teachings to serve as guidance for how to live with the changes that occur when practicing these sacred teachings. While this approach to teaching ancient Taoist practices may be considered modern, I have chosen to retain some Taoist words to describe different qualities of our sensual energy in order to expand both our understanding of our sensual selves and our vocabulary to describe it. I have also included a glossary at the back of this book clarifying the pronunciation and meaning of these Taoist words.

The Jade Goddess teachings address every aspect of our Feminine, including:

⟡ the physical: improving pelvic health, tone and suppleness

⟡ the emotional: healing wounds of past trauma

⟡ the mental: accessing limiting beliefs and replacing them with **life-enhancing** ones

⟡ the spiritual: connecting with the Divine Feminine essence.

Through many years of sharing with women the Jade Goddess teachings and the Art of Succulent Living, I have acquired an intimate understanding of women, their sensual natures, and how powerfully transformative these practices truly are. Within my classes, I have successfully instructed doctors, nurses, psychologists, counselors, PhD's, teachers, authors, mothers and women of all ages, backgrounds and experience. The core sentiment from all my students has been gratitude for the new understanding and experience of their sexual/sensual selves as it is integrated into their daily lives.

Developing Our Sensual Self and Awakening Our Life Force (Jing)

To effectively express our sensual self and understand how these ancient practices work, we need to understand how to awaken our innate life force (also known as Jing). Jing is found in our kidneys and is responsible for our natural libido and orgasmic experiences. All Taoist practices, including the Jade Goddess teachings, focus on nurturing our Jing for better health, longevity and greater orgasmic experience. As stated by Mantak Chia, "The kidneys store our sexual and energetic essences and purify the blood. The kidney center is called the Door of Life because it is also the center of Prenatal Chi, our inborn vitality."

Jing refers both to the *inherited* or *prenatal chi* (the energy created when the sperm and egg meet to form a human being) and *acquired* Jing (the energy taken in through air, food and positive life experience). This life force is the *vitality* that animates life in our body. Without it, we say that a person is deceased. Accessing and cultivating our Jing energy is one of the core Jade Goddess teachings. Sexual qi gong teaches us to conserve our *original* Jing while activating, cultivating and circulating our *acquired* Jing. This way, we can become more alive and sensual, while accelerating our evolution as human beings and attaining higher levels of self-mastery.

The Jade Goddess teachings cultivate Jing initially through the Taoist foundational practices. These practices (discussed in Chapter 7) are the essential groundwork we use to access and integrate succulence into our daily life. In addition, they also provide us with greater understanding and mastery of all our internal energies. By understanding how this life force works, we can direct it in creative ways to consciously increase vitality rather than deplete it. This ability to increase vitality, pleasure, ease and radiance within us is all part of the practice of the Art of Succulent Living.

The wondrous mystery and exploration of our bliss and ecstasy are not a passing fancy. They are our natural birthright as women. Through combining our knowledge with practical techniques, we embody our sensuality with the courage to live in a world that may not yet fully accept the Feminine. Now is the time for us to emerge as sensual women.

CHAPTER TWO

Succulence in a Barren World

The Philosophy Behind
the Art of Succulent Living

Sweet delightful
vibrations
move in fluid waves thru my body

rippling
opening
thrilling my every cell

as I remember you
alive and juicy
my body radiates her
exuberance to all around

the bliss of exploding ecstasy
spirals and spirals and spirals
'til I scream out in a gasp

around and around
your glorious presence
deep inside me dances
pushes, pulsates
in electric circles

please don't stop
dive into my soul

I am open
I am free
I am yours

OUR JOURNEY OF EMERGING AS SENSUAL WOMEN begins with the recognition of our birthright, and continues with the understanding of our relationship to the world around us. The Masculine is represented through our relationship to the men in our lives, whereas the Feminine, is represented through our sisterhood with other women. In order to reclaim our wholeness, we turn our attention inwardly and renew our commitment to our sensual selves. Through the lens of our sensuality, we can examine our lives with renewed dedication to our own evolution and empowerment.

Interactions with Men are Opportunities for Empowerment

Many women who desire to attract the attention of men through their sexuality often exhibit an interesting reaction. When men display arousal as a result of being stimulated by their succulence, it is common for these women to experience rage. The Jade Goddess teachings address this rage and acknowledge it as being simply an imbalance. As sensual women responding to the fullness of a man's interest, we can consider a new possibility beyond the reaction of anger. Our anger often stems from fear. These emotions, however, can be transformed through the practice of compassion and calmness. We can achieve this by breathing deeply into ourselves and realizing that beyond the perverse expression of arousal lies the Divine Masculine energy. When a man feels aroused, he is simply responding to our innate, awakened Divine Feminine energy. A healing and sacred exchange between individuals naturally occurs when we relax and allow ourselves to feel secure in our sensual nature. It is not necessary for both parties to be aware of this exchange between the Feminine and Masculine energies. In fact, all that is needed is for us to know that we personally do not have to do anything with anyone's response to our succulence.

STORY: *Walking in power*

One day, I chose to experiment with the effects of my outward sexuality while walking near Broadway in New York City. I was feeling lusciously vibrant and joyous. As I walked, I was aware of choosing to be in a place of celebration of all that came my way, including the bothersome catcalls, whistles, and comments. On this day I chose to make eye contact with those who were responding to my succulence. I sent out the understanding of what they were responding to and the fact that I accepted myself fully as a sensual woman. I found myself saying inwardly, "You like my butt, hair, whatever. Great! So do I! I love being admired as a sensual woman!" This lead to very interesting responses; instead of anger or aggression, I felt only gentleness and joy emanating from these men. It was an enlightening lesson in the power of celebration and sharing.

Exercise: Centering

This exercise returns us to our power center. It is especially useful when we find ourselves in a situation where we notice that a person is directing their attention and sexual excitement towards us.

The first step to transforming a situation into an empowering one is to take a moment to connect inwardly through simply *slowing down our breath.*

Once we shift our awareness inwards, we are able to notice how we are feeling. Feelings are important as they guide us towards greater compassion and security. Anger, fear, excitement, or any feeling beyond peacefulness and calmness is a strong reminder for us to center ourselves and to begin to create a greater sense of safety, peacefulness and calmness.

Exercise: Celebration Ceremony

This exercise creates greater ease and comfort when dealing with the attention of others.

As we breathe deeply into our belly, imagine that a person's attention is a celebration of our beauty. We do not have to look at the person, talk to the person, or interact on any level with that person. We do not have to respond to this person in any way. Simply thanking them inwardly for celebrating us is enough.

If we acknowledge an aroused person from a distance, it is easier for us to recognize arousal as a natural **Divine** response to aliveness. This *celebration ceremony* transforms our feelings of insecurity and apprehension into feelings of power and awareness. If we remember to follow our breath back into our center, we strengthen our ability to take our power back and make choices that inspire us to radiate a healthy glow of self-acceptance and self-confidence.

When we feel our succulence and live as sensual women, it is natural to draw attention to ourselves. Our innate aliveness is magnetic and does not require us to have that perfect body, to be young and slender, or to be wearing the latest fashions. All we require to live as sensual women is to feel our own succulence—and when we do, the world responds. Our challenge is to allow our beauty to shine as a gift without allowing external responses to shut down our vitality.

The key to this lies in our compassion and in understanding how our culture conditions men to behave in certain ways when a woman arouses them. If we judge this behavior, we limit our capacity to share our compassion. But if we look beyond the right or wrong and peer into the truth, there is space for us to choose the most empowering action. This truth is different for all of us, for as we progress on our path to living a succulent life, we will encounter many layers of truth. The most important lesson we can learn is to honor our inner guidance and to make our choices based on love and not fear.

Questions: Do you judge yourself or others for being sensual? How do you judge others for responding to your sensuality?

Interactions with Other Women are Intrinsic to Living as Sensual Women

Now that we understand our environment and how to transform the attention of men into empowerment, let's look at our connection to the women in our lives. As women, we naturally understand things about other women as we all share the common experiences of menstruation, pregnancy, beauty issues, and myths about men. According to a study done at UCLA, researchers found that the hormone **oxytocin**—fondly called the love hormone—is important for enhancing trust and reducing stress and that it is released when women spend time with each other. Dr. Laura Cousino Klein and researcher Shelley Taylor explain, "This encourages a woman to tend to children or seek the company of other women, and when she is so engaged, more oxytocin is released—which counters stress and has a calming effect." Therefore, cultivating sisterhood, the supportive bond between women, is part of a sensual woman's prescription to better health and less stress.

Sisterhood cultivates unconditional love and understanding through providing a social setting where there is a common understanding of what it means to be a woman. When we avoid women or create animosity with them, not only do we eliminate the possibility for experiencing genuine support, we also reduce the opportunity to nurture each other's essential feminine qualities: sharing, caring, and loving. Thus, being able to look at another woman as a sister and admire her instead of diminishing her, to celebrate her instead of criticizing her, is cultivating sisterhood.

In truth, we treat other women much like our inner voice treats us. Most women will admit that their inner dialogue is far from sweet, tender and supportive. Catty judgments and open disapproval of others is a reflection of our own inner dialogue. If we unconditionally accept ourselves, love every imperfection fully, and celebrate all of our endeavors, we will naturally radiate this beauty outward to all women. Simply put, how we see and treat ourselves is how we see and treat others.

Questions: Do you spend quality time with other women? What does your inner dialogue say to you?

Exercise: Transforming the inner dialogue

This exercise empowers our own self-image and enables us to access our genuine acceptance of other women.

Let's take a moment now to listen to our inner dialogue by first taking a few deep breaths and letting them out slowly. Once our breathing is calm, we become aware of our inner voice and can notice the constant chatter of our mind. What is it saying? Is it critical? Fearful? Wrathful? Or loving, supportive, and filled with celebration?

The next time we are around another woman, we can take a moment to go within and really listen to the monologue inside. What is its tone? Is it closed and critical or open and accepting? The more we pay attention to our inner dialogue from a place of neutral awareness and acceptance, the more we have the power to choose our feelings, our thoughts, and our experiences in the world. The ability to design our life as we choose is an act of self-empowerment.

Healing through Self-Acceptance

This process of transforming our inner dialogue gets easier as we become more conscious of our insecurity and self-loathing. These patterns are deeply ingrained within all of us making re-patterning ourselves as open, ecstatic beings of bliss a challenging part of emerging as sensual women. Each time we choose to release our judgment and share our radiance and love with others, we heal our hidden need to hide our darkness and failures, along with our light and successes. Living as sensual women begins with accepting ourselves in totality. Through self-love and self-acceptance we change our inner dialogue into a love language that shifts our perception of other women, transforming our critical lens into the lens of love and acceptance.

The Jade Goddess teachings help us to re-pattern ourselves by transforming our negative emotions into *virtues*. The more we become conscious of who we really are, the more we are able to compost the unnecessary and move into the fullness of living. These practices also help us access the ancient Taoist wisdom of the co-existence of **yin** with **yang**, of bad/negative with good/positive. This good/bad concept can be further understood by examining how perceiving a situation or person as "good" requires a simultaneous idea of a "bad" person or situation. So long as we judge—that is, make something good or bad—we will continue to separate our world into right and wrong. Yin and yang cannot exist in the absence of the other as they represent the two aspects of the whole. We experience this wholeness when we have total acceptance of our world.

Non-judgment is the key to perceiving others and our world with delight and wonderment and is the power of our awareness and choice. Our power is simply our ability to act. Through transforming our useless, negative patterns, we embrace our fellow sisters and ourselves as sensual women.

Questions: *Do you perceive the world through the lens of good/bad and right/wrong? How would using the perception of wholeness and acceptance change your view on life?*

Exercise: Vision for a benevolent world

This is a healing vision to initiate a shift in our connections with women.

Imagine a community where we women come together to dance, sing, cry, scream, and express ourselves fully without fear of judgment. Imagine every woman we meet understands our common bond of sisterhood and celebrates with us our unique beauty and success. Imagine a world where we celebrate and honor our partnership boundaries and transform our possessiveness into the healing energy of grounded love and self-assurance.

Empowerment Through the Feminine and Masculine

As children, our sensual little selves were enchanted by magical realms and often puzzled by the logic of grown-ups. Now as adults we seek comfort in our logic while remaining ignorant and fearful of the mystery of the magical. The Taoists are also aware of the dichotomy between magic and logic. But they view it as the *known* and the *unknown*, associating the *known* with yang (logical, clear, concise, and easy to see and dissect) and the *unknown* with yin (mysterious, intuition, synchronicity, unseen, and magical). So what happens when societies begin to shun magic and embrace logic? When societies become overly dependent on the yang and view logic as the only valid way of thinking, the result is a barren world, dry of the succulence inherent in the feminine mystery. Through the use of yin, the intuitive, magical aspect of living, we can counterbalance the overly logical yang expression. This balancing of our masculine logic with our feminine mystery plays an important role in maintaining our harmony both within us as individuals and within the lives we live. If we understand this process of blending our yang with our yin, we will see that emerging as sensual women is the key to restoring the balance of our modern day world and as we transform the barren world by healing our relationship to both the Masculine and the Feminine, we can in turn continue this healing by exploring the wisdom of both the known and unknown.

"Life is a mystery. A mystery so awesome that we insulate ourselves from its intensity. To numb our fear of the unknown we desensitize ourselves to the miracle of living."

— TIMOTHY FREKE

As sensual women, our calling is to embrace all of our desensitized parts and reawaken them. We open ourselves to our intuitive yin and harmonize it with our logical yang mind. Our emergence into the world as whole, integrated, sensual women includes being open to the magical. We say something is magical when we have no logical explanation for it. But does this mean the magical is less valuable than what is logically understood?

STORY: The power of the unknown

It had been over a decade since I had lost contact with my friend. Then, one week, I decided to look for him and I managed to connect with the mutual friend who had originally introduced us, but he had no idea where to find him. Several days later, I was visiting a small town about two hours from where I lived, and I happened to walk into a restaurant at the exact same moment that my old friend did. It was magical! Both of us stood in awe and excitement of the reconnection. Finally we laughed and hugged, and I shared with him my process of looking for him and how perfect it was that he was now standing in front of me. It felt as though no time had past between us, and we proceeded to exchange phone numbers and then go our own way.

STORY: The mystery of the unknown

It was 7pm on a Thursday night. I had a ticket for a seminar that I had purchased six months prior. The seminar was starting early the next morning. I had been to so many workshops, I simply could not go to another one.

I needed a weekend off, but I did not want to lose my money. So I put it out to the Universe: "Please, if there is any way someone else can use this ticket and I can get my money back, then let that happen now." Five minutes later, the phone rang. It was a wrong number, but since it happened immediately after my request, I decided to ask the person if she was going to the seminar tomorrow. She answered: "Yes! And I have a friend looking to buy a ticket too." I told her that I had a ticket and wanted to sell it. She said she'd call her friend, and within an hour, I was talking to her and we arranged to meet the next morning at the seminar. She got a ticket and I got the weekend off!

I shared these two stories to demonstrate the power of the unknown. Some may say it is coincidence or synchronicity. Whatever we choose to label it, for me, it was magic—the unknown at work. In the logical world, such things would not happen, and yet they did. Since beginning my journey practicing the Art of Succulent Living and the teachings of the Jade Goddess, I have had many such experiences of the unknown in my life. I would think a particular thought, and then moments later, there it would be, fully manifested exactly as I had imagined.

Questions: Do you believe in magic? Have there been times in your life where something purely illogical yet important and helpful occurred?

Our ability to manifest our thoughts becomes more and more powerful as we hone our sexual (creative) energy. This connection between cultivating our creative life force and harnessing and channeling our refined emotions and logical thoughts results in the ability to manifest. In addition, cultivating of our inner selves balances our lives by helping our logical mind relax and work with, instead of against, our intuition.

When we succeed to reunite our yin with our yang, our everyday world becomes sprinkled with magic. This magic is not just for children. It is also for the big kids who have forgotten that they are simply children who grew up and started calling themselves adults.

Our life contains within it every ingredient necessary to create whatever it is that we want. The problem is that most of us know what we don't want; thus, this is what we end up creating: what we don't want. We are always *creating*, whether we create what we want or don't want depends on how skillful we are at blending our logic with our intuition.

Exercise: Manifesting exactly what we want

Use to transform our: "I don't want" into "I choose".

Let us reframe this pattern of "I don't want" into the creative habit of choosing what we do want. For most of us, it is clear what we don't want in our life. Whatever we focus on, we get. If we focus on what we don't want, we get what we don't want. Let's take a moment to think of what we really do want in our life, then we can clearly state or write: "I choose this, that, or the other". For every "I don't want" statement, follow through with three "I choose..." statements.

If this exercise seems trite, let's pause for a moment and allow ourselves to just breathe in these ideas without needing to make them right or wrong. A part of ourselves may begin to feel lighter, perhaps even resonate with joy. This is the joy that comes to our spirit when there is no reason to laugh, we just do, when there is no reason to play instead of work, we just do, and when there is no reason to experience **orgasm**, we just do. We defy our logical mind by accepting that both logic and magic live together inside of us. Both deserve equal acknowledgement and both have their time and place. Let's celebrate the logic and magic that coexist within us as we cultivate and nourish our succulent lives.

> *Questions: When was the last time you did something that filled you with delight for no reason at all? Have you allowed yourself to be "un"-reasonable today? Have you smiled at someone you never smile at? Have you spontaneously bought flowers for yourself or a friend, or called someone with whom you haven't connected with for some time? Have you done anything that is "out of routine" or the "out of the ordinary" today?*

Our fear of the unusual and unknown may lead us to believe that a part of us is wrong or bad. Knowing we have the power to change our judgments, we can begin to embrace the illogical, unreasonable aspects of ourselves and relax into our fullness. When we are relaxed, our fears dissolve—we are no longer capable of being defensive or afraid. This is when we truly start to live, unafraid of who we really are and of how we manifest ourselves in this world. This is the Art of Succulent Living.

> *Question: Are you willing to risk appearing flaky, or silly, or crazy for the sake of allowing yourself the genuine experience of being alive?*

Exercise: Affirmation to embrace the totality of who we are

Take a few moments now to repeat the following (or design your own):

"I love myself exactly as I am right now. I am free to BE who I really am and who I really am is a beautiful, joyous, alive, succulent woman with infinite creativity, power, and bliss."

Some believe we only live once and if this is indeed true, then why inhibit our essential selves? Why waste another moment in fear instead of love? Why expend our vital energy being angry or depressed when we can channel it into ecstasy and joy? These are all important questions to consider as we allow our sensual self to emerge.

Reclaiming Our Virginity

Now that we have greater freedom in our personal expression by interweaving our masculine with our feminine wisdom, we can examine another area that greatly affects how we view ourselves as sexual beings, the concept of virginity. It is common for us to accept that our virginity is something that is lost and never to be reclaimed. The traditional and socially accepted definition of virginity is "a person who has not experienced sexual intercourse". The other definition describes virginity as being "in a **natural** or **pure** state". This implies that after experiencing sexual intercourse we no longer are in a natural or pure state, hence most of us believe sexual conversations and activities are "dirty".

When we examine the common description for sexual intercourse, we find the word **coitus** meaning "physical union of male and female sexual organs, leading to orgasm and ejaculation of semen". It is interesting to see that our traditional definition of virginity is not having experienced sexual intercourse. Does this mean that penetration of a finger or a dildo leaves a woman's virginity intact? These definitions also imply that intercourse or coitus is the physical union of male and female sexual organs, thus leaving out all same-sex acts of physical union. That would mean we have a large number of sexually active lesbian women (those who have never had sexual intercourse with a man) and gay men (those who have never had sexual intercourse with a woman) labeled as virgins! According to the descriptions above, we can only lose our virginity if we are with a member of the opposite sex, if there is orgasm (although it is not clear for whom), and if there is semen ejaculated. That leaves a lot of windows open, after all, not every sexual exchange leads to orgasm or to the ejaculation of semen.

Understanding how we define ourselves is valuable when we are seeking to redefine our relationship to both our sexuality and the world we interact with. Let us now investigate the word "virgin" from the second perspective, being "in a natural or pure state". To be natural and pure, a virgin would have to be:

- ✧ free from pretension
- ✧ spontaneous
- ✧ faithfully representing life

- ✧ free from contamination or foreign elements
- ✧ contain only that which is appropriate and be complete

In other words, virgins are women who are real (unpretentious), who are spontaneous (rather than regimented), who are complete or whole unto themselves, and who, with the purification practices of the Jade Goddess teachings, clear all contaminations and/or foreign elements/energies from their bodies. In this case, all sensual women who practice conscious sexual activity may consider themselves to be eternal virgins.

> *Questions: In light of this new information, how has your view of your own virginity changed? Do you consider yourself to be a virgin? Why or why not?*

Having only our own energy or chi within us is being truly *virginal*. So every time we make love, if we energetically cleanse ourselves afterwards, we can return to our natural virginal state of being. This is how we can maintain our virginity. No one can ever touch our essence—it is always pure, free, and willing to inundate all that we choose to create in our life. As we reclaim our virginity, we return to our innate sense of self. Through redefining ourselves according to our own truth and not according to what others lead us to believe, we deepen our trust in really knowing what is real for us.

Exercise: Connecting to our inner guidance

This exercise enhances our connection to our inner voice.

Let's take a moment now to close our eyes, breathe deeply into our belly, and relax into the exquisite sensation of breathing. Placing our awareness on where we are we become aware of all of ourselves. This connects us with our inner wisdom that lives within us and gives this wisdom both a voice and opportunity to be heard. Every moment of our life, we can check in with this inner guidance. When we do, we will know what is real and true for us. We know because it feels right, good, and natural.

Walking Away from Those We Love

Now that we have embraced the challenges of stimulating responses from the world around us, integrated our masculine logic with our feminine intuition, and remain ever fresh to the present moment, we can now allow ourselves the strength and compassion to look at our most potent challenge: leaving those we love. In life, there are times when those we love will not understand who we are at the profound level we desire. Our very succulence may even be a threat to them, and we may feel a temptation to regress back to our old shutdown, fear-based selves, afraid of not being loved. It is true that if we fully manifest our succulence, we may become unbearable to be near. But this is only because our very aliveness enables others to see their own deadness, their own lack of living life fully. This revelation is felt when they contact our aliveness, and this may threaten their very existence, or at least the existence of a fear-based **ego**. Naturally, it is too painful to see what is hidden, so instead of looking at what is revealed, their first instinct is to shut off our bright source of light that is shining upon their wounds.

In these times, all we can do as sensual women is bless our upset loved ones with our love, gentleness and compassion. If there comes a time when we must choose between being who we really are and losing a loved one (that is, keeping our connection to this person at the cost of our own truth), then we must approach this moment carefully for it will be a crucially defining moment. In considering these choices, we must remember that we can never change anyone. Ever. All we can do is change ourselves. Loving and accepting ourselves as we evolve and making positive, life-enhancing choices will allow our wisdom to speak clearly. Questioning the choices of others is not only disrespectful, it also asks them to justify their feelings. When desiring to respect both our own and other's choices, we would be wise to remember to live and let live.

Accepting differences in life choices can lead in one of two directions: living with others in harmony or realizing that the highest good for everyone involved would be through leaving the relationship. Once it is evident that our choice is to move on, to preserve our own integrity and aliveness, we will face the challenge of emotional pain, in ourselves and in the ones we love. Although walking away can be painful, it only hurts as long as we hold on to the confusion. Once we allow ourselves to breathe deeply and remember that our love and vitality is all we have to offer, a new moment is born. New opportunities for expansion and beauty present themselves every moment of our lives. When we die, it is our past that dies. But when we are reborn, a new moment, ripe for living, is born.

Questions: Are you currently in a situation that challenges your freedom and succulence? Are you willing to be accused of betrayal in order to honor your own inner voice and truth?

Exercise: Choosing to empower ourselves
This exercise helps us get more comfortable with making major life decisions.
    When we are faced with a decision to leave a loved one, we are wise to take a moment to feel deeply this experience. Through imagining what it

would be like we can confront our fears and doubts and transform them into renewed dedication to living our lives as fully as we can. Let's imagine ourselves making these difficult choices right now and allow ourselves to explore our feelings around living with these choices.

When we are open and free to shine our light unconditionally, we do not worry if others cannot love and accept us as we are, and we realize that loving and accepting ourselves as we are is more than enough. Our only real pain comes from making choices based on fear, limitation, and conforming to society's idea of the Feminine. Our healing comes with radiating our love and remaining open and loving even in the face of all that isn't love. As sensual women, we align ourselves with love and succulence, allowing our lives to become a wonderful dance filled with opportunity after opportunity to love more and to fulfill our succulent lives. This strengthens us in ways we have not yet dreamed of. Practicing the Art of Succulent Living in every moment is trusting our love and our succulence and giving it the space to really express itself and guide us. By this act, we will allow the succulence of our feminine wisdom to finally flow into this barren world.

CHAPTER QUESTIONS

Consider each of the following principles:
- ✧ succulent living
- ✧ magic
- ✧ fearlessness
- ✧ newfound virginity
- ✧ self-trust

How does each fit into your own life?

Does practicing the Art of Succulent Living bring up any emotions for you? What are they?

Are you willing to trust your inner wisdom and guidance above all else? Why or why not?

CHAPTER THREE

Integrity and Power

Compassion's Role
in Our Emergence

Beauty
beholds
you
smiling
deep into
those places
you refuse to look
or even love
shining herself
in and through
illuminating
activating
giving you
the strength
to be
ALL
that you are
now

W E CAN ENHANCE OUR AWARENESS of how we affect our world with our succulent nature by examining the importance of refining our integrity and power. If we redefine ourselves as sensual women, we must understand the complex roles that integrity and power play as we allow our sensual selves to emerge. If we practice both the teachings of the Jade Goddess and the Art of Succulent Living, we naturally feel an increase in our own personal power. Our challenge is to embrace this increase in our power while balancing it with the development of our integrity. This union of our power and integrity are the ingredients for developing our compassion chi.

Integrity: The Dance of Who We Are

The word integrity implies that which is integral or necessary to maintain life. Imagine our truth (spoken or unspoken) as being the glue that binds us to our core. The more we honor that truth, the more we are in contact with our core. Conversely, the less we recognize our truth, the further away we move from the essence of who we are. Integrity is living by our own truth while remaining in alignment with the greatest good of humanity. It means honoring all aspects of ourselves while living honestly, in wholeness and in harmony with others. It also means speaking our truth with love and power, without needing to be right or wrong, and living by our inner guidance and honoring life as it is. Finally, it means risking the loss of everything for the sake of maintaining our own authenticity.

Questions: How harmonious are you inside and out? Do you always speak your truth? If not, why not?

Exercise: Identifying our integrity
Identifying our integrity is valuable if we are to live in accordance with it.

An easy way to experience our integrity is to be silent for a moment and to allow ourselves to notice first how our body is feeling, then to notice both our emotions and our mind. When we feel our body relaxed, our emotions peaceful, and our mind restful, they are in alignment. Afterwards, it is a simple matter of noticing our body, feelings and thoughts before making a choice and seeing if they are in alignment or not.

Integrity implies unity or being complete. When our body, emotion, mind and spirit all agree to a choice we are making, we can say we are in *alignment* with ourselves or in a state of acting in integrity. When we are in internal conflict, it is impossible for us to act with integrity. What our mind says is ok our hearts may deem as unsuitable.

The Art of Succulent Living along with the Jade Goddess teachings invites us to connect to our body, feelings and thoughts as well as our spirit. We practice listening to our inner voice, and we notice what our inner messages are. When we sense a no from any aspect of ourselves, we honor that no and, thus, develop our level of personal integrity. The more in alignment we are with all that we are (body-mind-emotion-spirit), the more whole or complete we become.

As sensual women, this wholeness gives us greater access to our self-love, self-trust and self-acceptance that in turn enables us to access greater amounts of succulence. A common noticeable shift when practicing with the Jade Egg is the sudden awareness of the connection between our heart and our genitals. The more in alignment our love chi and sexual chi become, the more alive and vibrant we feel. This alignment of heart and sex is a powerful example of integrity that leads us to consciously choose when and how we engage in sexual activity.

Power: Our Succulence in Action

Power is our ability to act. We may act in ways that are in alignment with our integrity or out of alignment with our integrity. Regardless of which, we must understand that power itself is not good or bad, but the intention that initiates our actions will directly affect our happiness and well-being. The way in which we act or express our power determines the quality of our life. By consciously connecting with our power, we then are free to direct this power in ways that enhance our life-force and—therefore, increase our level of succulence.

The Art of Succulent Living and Jade Goddess teachings not only cultivate our integrity, they encourage us to claim our power with consciousness. Every one has power and no one can take power from us, only we can choose to give it away. When we give away our power, we give away our succulence and vitality. Through practicing the Jade Goddess teachings, we feel more powerful as we align our body, emotions, mind and spirit with the cultivation of our essential sensual nature. We notice that we can feel our presence more fully, and that our choices have quicker results and effects. Furthermore, the practices show us that we are the sole creator of our experiences, and therefore, that we no longer need anything external. We learn to validate ourselves, to fill ourselves with unconditional love, and to provide for ourselves the sensuality and pleasure we desire.

Question: Does expressing your power support or inhibit you?

Integrity and Power Become Compassion

If integrity is living in alignment with all aspects of ourselves and power is our ability to act, then integrated power is *the ability to act when fully aligned with our deepest truth*. Understanding the concept of integrated power is essential for the development of a sensual woman. In terms of energy, integrity may be seen as *be*-ing or yin energy, whereas power may be seen as *do*-ing or yang energy. If we combine integrity/*be*-ing/yin with power/*do*-ing/yang, we can create harmony and balance within us.

The Art of Succulent Living encourages the development of every aspect of us, not just our sexuality. Developing our sexual abilities and prowess leads to greater power but this must be balanced by the development of our consciousness (awareness and integrity). To develop our consciousness we must learn how to open and activate our heart and learn to cultivate compassion.

"The more fulfilled you are sexually, emotionally, and spiritually, the more energy and joy you will have to share with everyone in your life."

— RACHEL ABRAMS

According to Mantak Chia, "with compassion, one can love unconditionally and thereby accept the world on its own terms without suffering." Taoists believe that our heart is the seat of our consciousness and accept that within our heart lives the potential for compassion and unconditional love as well as pure awareness. As sensual women, it is wise for us to be aware of our hearts as we become more magnetic due to having more sexual chi. It is common when first learning the practices of the Jade Goddess teachings for our ego to come into play through feelings of being better than others and through the desire to control others with this new magnetism. Energetically, this means that our sexual energy remains unrefined and may stay in our **solar plexus** when we do not consciously move our succulence up to our heart and higher centers.

We can tend to manipulate when we do not properly channel our sexual energy in our body such as with sexual meditations (Chapter 8, the sexual foundation practices). If there are any blockages in our body, our sexual energy will tend to stay stuck in those areas and amplify whatever the blockage is. For example, if there is anger in us and we do not cleanse our liver of this **stagnant chi**, we will grow more anger in ourselves or attract it into our life. The Taoists view the ego as being the lower emotions (anger, envy, fear, mistrust, jealousy) and the center for the lower emotions is the solar plexus. The key to preventing stagnation from occurring is to make certain that the energy of the heart is open and blending with the aroused sexual energy. If we focus on circulating our newly cultivated sexual energy while at the same time cultivating our virtues using the Jade Goddess teachings, we can focus our energy on developing the chi of compassion. Compassion chi is responsible for evolving our ego/solar plexus into a conscious, integrated and powerful will.

Question: How does compassion help us to balance our integrity and power?

Exercise: Smiling into compassion

This exercise helps to transform arousal into vitality.

Whenever we feel aroused, an exercise known as the inner smile (see the inner smile, Chapter 7), helps us transform and refine our sexual chi first into higher virtues, then finally into compassion. Here is how it works:

The next time we are aroused, let's take a few moments to smile inwardly and allow ourselves to feel relaxed, open, kind, gentle, courageous, and loving. As our arousal builds, we connect to our heart and allow the chi inside our heart to grow and transform into more compassion chi. We accomplish this simply by smiling inwardly.

As we practice refining our sexual energy, we begin to see how compassion plays a key role in developing our integrity and power in a harmonious way. This practice connects us directly to our heart, allowing our compassion chi to permeate our intentions. This is an essential part of developing more compassion and evolving our egos into higher will. If we do not remain mindful while refining our sexual chi, this chi will stagnate (remain in an unrefined state) and inhibit our access to our integrity and power. This is what leaves us with an activated ego.

A normal response to this form of inner stagnation is the activation of hidden desires and fears. Using this new power to get what we want—to control outcomes or people—is an act of misdirected chi and ego. It is precisely what we do not want to do when practicing the Art of Succulent Living. However, if we focus on developing our compassion, integrity and power simultaneously while developing our sexual chi, we can experience the alchemical fusion of orgasm and love—what I call **cum-passion** or compassion chi.

Compassion chi is created by opening a clear energetic path between our heart (fire/yang) and our **yoni**, the female genitals (water/yin) and by successfully balancing *be*-ing (integrity) with *do*-ing (power). This chi that flows between our fire (heart/love) and our water (yoni/orgasm) poles in our body creates a potent synergy between our two centers. Compassion thus enables us to access more integrity, more personal power, and more self-esteem.

With compassion, we understand that not everyone will be a master of their own sensual energy. When people react to our succulence we must remember we are the ones with the tools and the ability to make conscious choices that come from our compassionate intention. Sometimes this compassion may become fierce compassion, a passion that establishes clear and strong boundaries. Fierce compassion allows us to say no with love in our hearts to the demands of our lovers and then stand our ground in this choice without moving into our conditioned response of care-taking our partner's feelings.

Allowing people the freedom to react in whatever way they choose, while maintaining an open heart with powerful clarity, feels loving and freeing as it eliminates fear from the situation. As sensual women we learn this art of speaking our truth while practicing honoring our own boundaries and maintaining a compassionate heart. This act of compassion creates freedom and openness, allowing us to access more vitality and succulence. We see that being succulent is not just an act of being sweet and compromising—it is also an act of integrity and power.

Exercise: The quality of our intentions

This exercise helps us to develop our awareness of our intentions.

Next time we find ourselves in a situation where we are exchanging energy with another, let's notice where our intention is coming from. Is it coming from our belly? Our heart? Our mind? Do we feel a need to be right? Or better? Or stronger? Or sexier? Let's look to see if we need to feed our ego or if we desire to share our love and radiance?

The Beauty of Boundaries

Having boundaries does not mean having to put a brick wall around ourselves. It means maintaining a fluid and flexible awareness of our personal space. Fluid boundaries can expand and contract with our intention. Some situations might require keeping energy contained within, whereas other situations may require boundaries that are much more expansive.

Questions: What does having boundaries mean to you? How does the concept of a fluid boundary feel?

For many, the very idea of keeping a boundary feels like a limitation. We may feel that this limits the full potential of an experience. In one sense, this is indeed true, yet in another sense, having a container that has no leaks (clear boundaries) allows for more of the experience to be felt. How do boundaries interplay with integrity and power? Understanding boundaries will help identify situations where we are experiencing our actions (power) without being in alignment with our body-mind-spirit (integrity). Boundaries serve as a useful tool for cultivating both succulence and compassion.

Boundaries that stem from fear are usually created by our need for control. These types of boundaries protect us by keeping other energies out, but at the same time, they also limit us from experiencing events that could potentially transform us. On the other hand, when boundaries stem from compassion, an essence of freedom arises. This freedom allows us to feel conscious of all parts of ourselves in any given situation. If we do not know where we stand or where our thoughts and emotions are, then how can we be in integrity? Whether we choose to use our power to create a dance of control and self-protection, or we choose to activate our sense of presence and compassionate awareness, is ultimately an individual choice.

Questions: Do you create your boundaries from fear or compassion? How do your boundaries serve you?

When we, as sensual women, tap into our compassion to create fluid boundaries to live more authentically and with greater integrity, our inner and outer worlds become congruent. This ability to access compassion and bliss at will is the gift of fluid boundaries. This is the true meaning of power. Being powerful is different from having power over a situation or person. When we are fully conscious of our power (our ability to act) and we infuse that with our sensuality and love (compassion), we are able to act with integrity at any given moment.

When power is balanced by integrity and activated by compassion our sensual essence begins to thrive. While power can be seen as chi moving outwardly into the world, integrity can be seen as chi moving inwardly into the body-mind-spirit. Like the yin and yang, they co-exist more potently as a synergy than apart. This integrated synergy of compassion transforms the challenges of our life into an adventure of our full sensual emergence.

Exercise: Defining integrated power

This exercise identifies our own version of our integrity and power.

Let's write down a list of words that come to mind when we think of integrity, of power, and of living authentically. When we have finished our list, let's review it and define for ourselves, in our own words, what it means to live according to our inner truth. Afterwards, let's practice living our newly defined truth. When we forget, we can smile to ourselves with compassion and renew our choice to continue our efforts to live authentically.

Living with integrated power enhances our ability to choose. When life manifests a challenge it equally manifests the ability to transform the challenge into a gift. By breathing deeply, tuning into ourselves (*be*-ing), and then responding (*do*-ing), a harmonious expression of the authentic self emerges. Taking time out from situations to collect our thoughts and feelings and rooting ourselves deeply into the earth, enhances our personal power. That in turn enhances all of our life situations. We witness this integration through experiencing greater ease and inner peace within while becoming more effective as mature, loving women in society. To be powerful is to live with full understanding of our personal integrity and to consciously express this outwardly in the world as compassion.

CHAPTER QUESTIONS

Let's look again at the following relationships: Integrity as yin or be-ing and power as yang or do-ing. Can you relate to this way of understanding integrity and power? Why or why not?

What are your feelings on fluid boundaries and their effect on integrity and power?

How will this understanding of integrated power help you make choices in your life?

CHAPTER FOUR

Conscious Living

Awareness as the Key to Unlocking
Our Power and Succulence

Ride this river of eternal life
with me
see me laugh, see me cry
see me play your favorite song
on the wings of a dragonfly
take part in this adventure
set sail into the setting sun
chase your dreams
with abandon and trust
flow with this endless source
let go more than ever before
forget your name
free your soul
open your heart
and dare to love life fiercely
break free from
your tortured thoughts
watch them
drop like pebbles into the river bed
only to transform into grand rainbows
climb up high
slide down these iridescent bridges
into the reality of what you fully are.

As we cultivate compassion through the harmonious expression of our integrity and power, we further benefit through awakening our consciousness. The Art of Succulent Living harnesses this awareness to skillfully navigate through our conscious beginnings, conscious endings, and conscious choices. The use of our conscious awareness facilitates graceful resolution of our practical issues of living with the shifts and changes that come when we embark on our emergence as sensual women.

The Wisdom of Conscious Living

Our consciousness is our ability to be finely attuned and aware both internally and externally, and conscious living is our ability to navigate through our daily lives with this greater awareness. The practice of noticing our feelings, thoughts and bodily sensations activate our deeper awareness and allow us to delve into examining our choices and reactions to life's ever-changing situations. Therefore, to live consciously is more than just the mental process of understanding what is happening around us in a solely logical manner. It is also the ability to listen to the wisdom of our body, emotions and spirit.

> Questions: Are you aware of yourself fully? Do you know what is happening in your body right now? Do you feel connected to the source of all your emotions? Are you able to feel your own core truth (spirit)? What does that feel like? Which part of you makes all the decisions?

Practicing the Art of Succulent Living involves becoming aware of ourselves in every way; then, from this place of awareness, making choices that resonate with every aspect of who we are. The Jade Goddess teachings specifically cultivate deeper awareness of all aspects of ourselves. Through both practical and mental modifications, we can learn to cultivate our ability to be conscious and to be fully aware of our body-emotions-mind-spirit.

We know that acting from an integrated place means that we are not fighting ourselves. One core aspect of being conscious is working in harmony with all that we are. Here is an example of non-integrated living: we feel scared about having sex but justify the fear through logical thinking—for example, we think "this is what lovers do when they are together". Then we make a choice to have sex in that moment even though we are feeling totally shut down sexually. There are three types of messages to be aware of here: physical (un-aroused sexual energy), emotional (fear), and mental (sense of duty). The non-integrated choice is to have sex even when we are un-aroused, feeling fear, and creating logical reasons to ignore our emotions and the messages our body is trying to communicate.

Now let's take this same scenario and apply an example of integrated living. We are feeling scared and sexually un-aroused, but this time, we mentally check in with the source of those messages. By doing so, we determine that we feel a lack of trust in our partner. Knowing this, we are able to use these powerful messages to make a conscious choice not to have sex despite what our partner may want us to do or believe.

> *Questions: How does an integrated choice differ from a non-integrated choice? Recall times when you have both made integrated and non-integrated choices. What is your new understanding of the differences between the two types of choices?*

Another aspect of conscious living is the ability to exercise our awareness. When we exercise our awareness and act in an integrated way, we tap into something that is very powerful: our own ability to discern what it is we truly want from life. It is important to point out that sometimes we may have awareness of being out of integrity yet still consciously choose to act anyway. In such circumstances, we, as sensual women, are choosing to take full responsibility for our choices and the consequences that those choices bring. Sometimes going out of balance is in itself an act of staying in balance. When we do not allow ourselves to make mistakes, we prevent ourselves from embracing the full spectrum of our human experience.

As sensual women we are conscious of making mistakes, and we accept the consequences of our choices while allowing each experience to be free of judgment. By living in this dual state of non-judgment and conscious awareness, we are able to realize the perfection of every experience. As we explore our ability to make more conscious choices in our lives, we can enhance the perfection of who we are.

The Power of No

What is choice? When do we really have the power to choose? We have the power to choose when we choose to say no. When we learn how to say no we are choosing not to act out whatever we happen to be feeling without conscious consideration.

Our ability to say no is one of the powerful lessons explored through applying the wisdom the Art of Succulent Living and Jade Goddess teachings. In order for the energy of sexual exchange to be liberated from its dogma, karma, sin, heaviness, or negative charge, it must be handled with skillful awareness. This energy is a powerful and precious resource. Tapping into it can create everything from life (a baby) to whatever preoccupies our thoughts (such as, manifesting thoughts of being hurt, or finding a partner). It is better to become aware of our sexual energy, the fuel for our brain and thoughts, and use it, then let it run havoc in our life. By consciously cultivating and circulating our sexual energy, for example, we develop our awareness and understanding of our sexual natures. In this way, we have the power to consciously choose our sexual encounters instead of being a victim of our urges.

Questions: Have you exercised your power to say no lately? What is one thing that you feel you are willing to say no to?

By exercising the choice *not to do this or that,* we are then free *to do exactly this or that.* For example, if we drink alcohol and believe that we are doing this out of a conscious choice, then we can test our ability to choose through stopping our drinking of alcohol for a month. We consciously choose to stop. If we are unable to stop, or if we meet resistance, then we are not really choosing to drink alcohol; rather, we are acting out an addiction. If we are able to not drink alcohol and then we genuinely make the choice to start drinking it again, we are expressing our conscious power of choice.

Exercise: The power of choice

The next time we sense ourselves about to act out of habit, let's stop and see what it feels like to not go through with it. Instead, let's just sit and breathe the sensation of this choice, being aware of all our resistance patterns, logical justifications, and inner arguments that may arise.

When choosing to be more conscious in all areas of our life, the best way to start is with small, slow steps. The transition from living as though we have no choice (addictions/habits) to living knowing we always have a choice takes patience and compassion. The more we practice, the more confidence we will gain in living a conscious life. The motto from the martial art master Bruce Lee, "no limitation as limitation", helps us to open ourselves up to life's infinite possibilities. Life is a series of experiences, choices, and the creation of our desires, thoughts, emotions, etc. Living as sensual women means exercising our perception of limitless possibility while creating harmonious connections to the rest of the world.

Questions: How do you limit yourself? What would it be like for you to choose a limitless perception of life? Do you recognize your addictions?

A sensual woman views a limitation as a choice based on fear. These fear-based choices also lead to infinite possibilities yet there is the misconception that no other choice is available. All fear-based choices essentially imply a limit, and therefore, limitations are redefined to mean personal choices that are **life-taking** in nature. We can see fear-based choices as the act of moving away from what we want, whereas love-based choices are the act of moving towards what we want. Therefore, making freedom and loved-based choices becomes a life-giving experience. When a judgment of limitation is placed upon a life-giving experience, we can reorient our perception to understand this choice as one leading to expansion. For example, choosing to avoid processed sugars may be viewed as limiting, yet the choice is essentially *life-giving*, and therefore, can be perceived as a love-based choice.

> *Questions: Do you make choices based on fear or on freedom and love? Do you feel like you "have no other choice" in any area of your life? Do you judge other people for the choices they make in their lives? Do you attempt to impose your own "limited" beliefs on others?*

As sensual women we create limitless experiences for ourselves based on the belief that we are here to fully taste all that life has to offer. Living by this belief includes allowing others the same freedom. Therefore, the choice to limit another person or judge their choices loses its charm. Every choice leads to a multitude of other choices, and literally, there is an infinite web of possibilities to choose from.

If so many possibilities exist within all people, why then are we feeling limited or choosing to limit others? Living in the frequency of fear, we naturally fear the choices of others and experience a desire to control or make choices for them. Living in the frequency of love and freedom, we naturally rejoice in the infinite wealth of possibilities that exist for others. From a love-based life, fear is understood to have nothing to do with any person, place or thing, and everything to do with the choice to be in fear. As sensual women we view our fears as flags indicating where we have forgotten our innate love and freedom.

Exercise: Transforming fear into opportunity

This exercise helps us move from fear into love.

A simple formula for transforming fear is to feel deep gratitude. Practicing the Art of Succulent Living is choosing gratitude when fear is prevalent. This act of seeing when we have forgotten and returning to our own truth, our power, our center (core essence) or love (the universal vibration of creation) can and does set us free—free to experience our ultimate expression: who we really are now. Let's practice using this simple formula of transforming fear into gratitude as often as we can through always remembering what we are grateful for.

Bringing to Light Unconscious Power

Unconscious power manifests itself whenever we find ourselves in a position where we are able to manipulate the world without fully understanding how or why this process works. Unconscious use of our power to affect the world can lead us to creating things that are undesirable for ourselves, such as unwanted dynamics with others. There are essentially no advantages to this behavior, whereas the disadvantages can be compared to driving a car blindfolded. The chances of experiencing physical, emotional or psychological pain increase as does the impact of such activity on our families, friends and communities. An example of this would be when a woman attracts to her a married man and uses her magnetism to seduce him into an experience that may cost him his marriage.

Conscious power is our ability to act in synergy with our integrity. We use our conscious power to be fully aware of our abilities and to design our life according to the virtues we have chosen to hone. Compassion, the energy of our heart (love) merging with that of our genitals (orgasm), is one such virtue. This fusion of our polar energies of yang and yin, heaven and earth, fire and water, hot and cold, is a process of inner alchemy that activates our highest abilities. The heart without sexual energy is love without succulence; sex without the heart is passionless. They are perfectly designed for each other and when they are united, we experience our conscious power, the power that creates the succulent life we truly desire.

> Questions: Have you experienced love without sex or sex without love? What was it like? How do you think you would feel if you combined these two energies, if you merged sex and love?

Conscious Beginnings

What does it mean to consciously begin a relationship? Our ability to be clearly aware of our intentions at the start of any relationship happens through our understanding of the impulse that drew us to the person in the first place. Knowing this, we as sensual women can create from a place of integrated power. Understanding our impulses enables us to be aware of all of our reasons when we choose to initiate something new and is an invaluable tool in the arena of sexuality and relationships. In a sense, each day we are beginning anew our relationships with everyone; however, for the practicality of exploration, let us focus our attention on the impulse or desire that fuels the beginning of an intimate relationship.

Our understanding of our own personal impulses shifts us from feeling that we are victims claiming that it just happened to us, to empowered women aware of when these impulses move through us and when we are acting according to these impulses. This shift brings our consciousness into the present moment and gives us the freedom to genuinely choose whether or not to initiate an intimate relationship based on what we are noticing as our impulse. What is this impulse exactly? An impulse can come in many forms—that is, in the form of love, lust or procreative urges.

All three impulses (love, lust and procreative urges) are part of the human experience and are essential in their own right and time. In discussing conscious beginnings, we must be able to determine what is indeed influencing our choices. Only then can we act according to our highest potential. For example, if we realize that the sole reason for being so kind and open towards a person we just met is due to the intense amount of arousal/lust that is racing through our blood, then we can choose our actions accordingly. When we consciously choose to enter an intimate relationship with another individual, be it a few brief moments or a lifetime, it is helpful to clarify which influential impulse is active. None of our impulses are necessarily wrong, but if we do not know why we are choosing what we are choosing, then are we really making a choice? If we know our motivations as we begin our intimate relationships, we can have more conscious awareness and, therefore, more integrity and power in our connections.

Questions: Are you aware of your impulses? Recall a time when you initiated an intimate relationship and see if you can map out if love, lust or procreative urges, may have been the impulse to begin this connection. Can you see the value in creating beginnings from a conscious place?

Impulses of Love, Lust and Urges

Love. As we all know, there are many different shades of meaning for this word. For the sake of simplicity, let's define love as respect for another person. Love is also the constant opening of our heart and the willingness to experience life from this place. When our heart is broken or closed, we tend to say that we are no longer *in love*. So, in this case, to be *in love* is to have our hearts open at all times, even when it is painful to do so. The truest love requires no reason for its existence and is all-conditional; that is, it remains open to love no matter what condition the relationship is in. Love exists through our willing hearts.

Lust. Lust is our deep, primal desire to express our life force or sexual energy. When we are lustful, we feel it in our loins, a throbbing beacon of erotic drive. This is a powerful, passionate, and vivacious energy. True lust is wild, free of guilt, willing to fully express itself. Lust exists through our willing sex centers.

Essentially, the difference between love and lust lies in the nature of their energy. The chi of love is of the fire element and is stored and created in our heart center, whereas the chi of lust is of the water element and is stored in our kidneys and sexual center. Love is considered an impulse associated with refined energy, while lust is seen as an impulse associated with unrefined or raw energy. This does not mean that love is essentially better, it simply indicates that sexual energy or lust is a chi that we can refine as powerful fuel. Love can be experienced outside of a sexual context just as lust can be experienced outside of a love context. However, when we bring love and lust, fire and water elements together, we create a very powerful and healing synergy. Instead of viewing them as rivals, these two qualities when brought together consciously can create something greater then either energy expressed alone. Hence, they both play a vital role in our own inner alchemy and in the manifestation of compassion. Understanding the nature of love and lust individually allows us to map out where we are energetically.

> Questions: Which center are you more aware of? Are you aware of how these two centers activate individually at different times? What message are they sharing with you? Have you experienced the synergy of love and lust?

Procreative urges. This third impulse describes the state when all sense and reason are thrown out the door. This is *not* an issue of *love* or *lust*, but an issue of the body, more specifically one of our biological imperatives, our need to propagate. Richard Dawkins, author of *The Selfish Gene*, writes about how there is a relationship between our macrocosm and microcosm. He sees the connection between the DNA/genes (microcosm to reproduce itself) and the urge to get pregnant (macrocosm). His work helps us to understand how our behaviors and choices (macrocosm) may have possible links to inner chemical messages stored within our genes (microcosm). In essence, Dawkins leaves us pondering the possibilities that not all human impulses are obvious, and indeed, some impulses may be rooted in our very DNA. Therefore, if our genetics can have such a profound impact as to influence our choices, i.e. the necessity of genetic survival and thus, the urge for procreation, we may choose to examine our impulses with greater curiosity. As sensual women practicing the principles of the Art of Succulent Living, we have the opportunity to question our use of love and/or lust in moments of procreative urges (behaving unconsciously) and to begin to act with greater awareness of who we are. Procreative urges exist through our DNA.

This procreative urge is witnessed when a woman suddenly must have a baby! There is no logic to this and we jokingly call it the biological clock—and in a sense this is true. Our procreative urges, which stem from the survival messages of our genes, may bypass our conscious mind, and possibly create temporary behaviors (love and lust) to affect an outcome. This may sound gruesome, but really it is not. At what point does our consciousness kick in when we are inundated with intense procreative hormones? Hopefully before we act in ways that are not supportive to our growth.

> *Questions: Have there been times in your life when you have felt real love? Or true lust? Or procreative urges? Think about a time when you have felt a moment of intense desire to seek something even though there seemed to be no particular conscious reason for it.*

We will most likely not know when we are experiencing procreative urges because when we are, it is almost impossible to think about anything else. Our hormones may be working on a microscopic level, but that does not mean they are not powerful. So becoming conscious of their occurrence needs to happen prior to their occurring. If we find ourselves encouraging ejaculation in an unprotected exchange at our fertile time of month, we can take a moment or two (or three for some) to breathe deeply and center ourselves. Our ability to slow down and engage our conscious awareness can help us to eliminate a possible unwanted pregnancy.

When we find ourselves in a procreative urge, we can pause and ask ourselves sincerely "do I really want to do this" and "what are the consequences of these actions?" If our answer is yes and we are willing to fully accept the consequences of our choices (pregnancy), then this may well be an ideal (natural) time to be hormonally influenced. But if our answer is no (or yes to the first question, but we are not willing to accept the consequences), then we need to put on the brakes. This may be a great time for solo-cultivation—that is, a time for deep self-love and compassion—as we enter into a tough battle of wits versus hormones.

The best way I have found to balance myself is to do my healing sounds and to smile to every organ, making sure I am internally balanced. Nature walks are great. Exercise of any kind is fantastic. Wearing the Jade Egg also helps a lot.

Exercise: Transforming our impulses

*This exercise uses the foundation practice—the **micro-cosmic orbit**, where our tongue rests on the roof of our mouth to facilitate the flow of energy through our body (see both Chapter 7 and Chapter 11 for more information).*

If we are in the midst of a mega-dose of procreative hormones, remembering to breathe and bring that sensation into our orbit helps. Massaging our breasts and visualizing our hormones becoming more and more balanced is a powerful healing. These hormones are life-enhancing and circulating them through our orbit will create a sense of balance in the middle of the chaos. Youthful hormones are rejuvenating to our body and give us a healthy glow and a bounce to our step.

On my path of practicing the Art of Succulent Living, the most brilliant gift I have received is the Jade Goddess teachings and its practice. These practices have given me the power to choose in moments where I normally would not have been consciously aware enough to choose. When I am in the impulse of lust, I can wear my Jade Egg which helps me connect with the aroused energy in my genitals. Then I can circulate my aroused energy using the foundation practice of the micro-cosmic orbit to move the intensity of arousal away from my genitals to other parts of my body. I can still choose to flirt if I want to. What is important is that I am aware of my actions and why I am doing them. I have seen many people believe that they are in love when in reality they are in lust or even experiencing procreative urges.

We know when love is real because it feels natural. We feel at home and safe and willing. We feel like ourselves and do not feel the need to pretend to be anything different. We see the human side of our partner and respect them fully. We are in a place where fear does not come into play. When we sense our physical heart/chest area, it feels full and open. In that moment of pure love, we have the choice to either send it back deep inside all parts of our own being and smile in the acknowledgment that we are open in our heart center or we can choose to consciously share this heart opening.

The Art of Succulent Living empowers us to always be aware that the love we feel really does come from us and not another. However, we may choose with our partner to exchange this love energy and amplify the **love vibration** in each other. The love vibration or heart chi is a potent energy that we personalize into the love of oneself and the love of others. The feeling of love is simply the energy or vibration of the activated heart. In Taoist terms, this chi is also called the **imperial fire** and is vital in keeping other chi in the body activated as well as playing a part in the inner alchemy of transforming raw sexual energy into compassion. Thus activating love in the heart is healing for the body-mind-spirit and it feels like openness, natural joy and expansion. The true gift of conscious love is when it is used to enhance both our own and our partner's evolution.

Fear and doubt are not a part of love. They are the parts of us that need love. So if we find ourselves feeling the incredible bliss of love pulsating through our body, we share this true blessing with ourselves first. We gift ourselves with this healing elixir. When we feel full and centered, we share it with not only our chosen love, but all of life. Let's shine the radiance of our heart onto the world. We and all whom we touch will be enriched by it.

Questions: When you are "in love", are you able to give yourself the love you feel for your partner? Are you afraid of what would happen if they were no longer in your life?

We know when we are in lust because it feels like a thick, raw passion that is throbbing so hard in our sex center that it may even be mildly uncomfortable. This discomfort is what really tends to motivate us to act on our lust because we want to be released from it. So we act out in ways that we feel will help us literally release the tension that lust has created in our body.

When lust comes out to play, we have the opportunity to not judge it or label it as wrong, dirty, or fearful. Instead, we can breathe into our aching yoni and smile the warmth of our heart down into her. We can enjoy the intensity of this sensation and encourage it to move into our orbit, allowing our whole body to experience this aliveness. The key is to first share our lust with ourselves and feed the parts of us that are yearning to be touched and honored. Once we feel full and very juicy, then we can choose to share this with another, better yet with all of life.

While lust has gained a more negative reputation than its counterpart, love, we can consider it to be no less revered for it is a very natural and innate expression of life. For example, in the spring we see a rise in lust in the world around us. We call it spring fever. If we can accept this phenomenon in nature, why do we find it so hard to accept it in ourselves? The next time we choose to share our lust with another, let's be very conscious of what form of agreement we make with this person. Let's not use another as a tension releaser. We have our own practice to do that and we can cultivate this powerful energy while taking care not to dissipate it or repress it. Dissipating it will only deplete our chi while repressing it will create congestion of chi in the body. By honoring our lust, it will reward both our partner and ourselves with its rejuvenating and creative properties.

Questions: When you feel lust, do you feel overwhelmed by it or do you enjoy it? What is your relationship with this primal power?

We can choose to view sex as a very natural, integral part of the human experience. Understanding that sex is not any more special than the other ways in which we choose to experience life changes it into one of the many choices we have to express ourselves in the world. Also, by viewing our expression of pleasure as permeating all of our physical activity, such as eating, defecating, sleeping and exercising, we invite the possibility of orgasm into every instant of our life. Conscious orgasm is a matter of choice, not a matter of arousal or sex. The knowledge that we do not need sex to experience orgasm allows sex to settle into an equal status with all other physical experiences.

Questions: How do you view sex in comparison to all other human functions? How does sex fit into your idea of yourself?

The understanding that sex is a natural, normal part of our life frees us as sensual women to understand that we no longer need sex to experience the pleasure of orgasm. However, if we do choose to share in this delicious energy, by all means let's enjoy it fully. Remember, in order to do this, both partners must be consciously aware of this agreement. For example, when I would choose a partner just for the purpose of exchange (not because I'm in love or want to reproduce), I would let them know beforehand. Normally, people are very open to this and are often relieved to know our inner thoughts. This sharing creates a freedom in which we both can fully enjoy and play in the wonderful creative force of raw sexual passion.

Exercise: Activating our throat center

This exercise helps us speak honestly about our impulses and desires, while strengthening our ability to make conscious choices.

We can either practice the following sample quotes or write our own words to express our truth.

"I am interested in enjoying fun, sensual play with you. I would like to know how you feel about this?

"I am a woman making choices to fully express my sexuality in healthy ways and I am not interested in manipulating you or in making more of this connection. I just want to have a fun experience of sex with no strings attached and would like to know how you feel about this."

Question: How does the idea of expressing your desire authentically and openly feel to you?

Tips for Conscious Sexual Choices

When we embark in being conscious about our sexual choices we must realize that some people are very open to the invitation while others are not. Some people feel they need to be in a committed relationship before they can open up sexually. It is important to communicate clearly what our desires are as well as what our intentions are when we initiate a sexual relationship. Occasionally, we may find that people are interested in becoming our practice friend or lover. This works when both parties are clear from the beginning what their intentions are. If this is the case for us, we must remember to check in constantly to see if there has been any changes or shifts within this intention.

Question: How does the idea of having a practice/play friend feel to you?

Power of Three

I have found that three is the magical number when it comes to sexual exchanges. With less than three exchanges we tend to call the connection casual. With more than three sexual exchanges new expectations can begin to form. This is also known as **sexual bonding**. Sexual bonding simply means a connection that is more potent than just a casual experience. For example, when friends have an adventure together, they might refer to it as their bonding time. This does not imply that sexual bonding is a long-term commitment or a form of bondage. To minimize sexual bonding, we can constantly remind our lovers that each time is a first time and it may not imply that there will be a next.

> *Questions: How does the idea of bonding in casual sex feel to you? Does being more conscious and open about your needs create fear? Apprehension? Anger? Disgust? Joy?*

By making a conscious mutual agreement, we are also able to benefit from the refinement of raw sexual chi. This refining process is possible through using the micro-cosmic orbit, one of the key foundation practices of the Art of Succulent Living. When we feel our raw sexual energy, we can move it through our orbit and refine it. This refinement helps us create a sacred communion of two lusty adults, free of guilt, purely manifesting themselves in the now. This is very potent and healing. Many people enter casual sexual experiences because they think they are lustful, when really they are looking to be **lust-full**, that is, to be filled by another's lust.

If we enter into these lust-full experiences because we feel the need to be socially accepted or to feel beautiful and loved, we must remember the truth of these unconscious exchanges most often leave us feeling emptier than not. So as we play more consciously when lust comes about, we can enjoy it, cultivate it, circulate it, and share in the celebration of this vibrant, glowing magnetism that naturally exists between two sensual, sexual beings. As sensual women, offering our sexual energy and yoni is a sacred gift, to be shared with discernment and wisdom.

> *Question: Can you recall a time where you did something sexual and later questioned yourself with thoughts like 'What was I thinking?!' or 'I can't believe I just did that!'?*

A powerful aspect of practicing the Art of Succulent Living is consciously knowing why and when we are choosing love, lust, or procreation (or, as some say, recreation) when we engage in sexual exchange. As I mentioned before, all of these are not bad reasons for sexual communion. In fact, it is not really the reason that I want to bring attention to such impulses. When we know ourselves intimately, we can then choose wisely. This way, instead of feeling confused by our choices, we gain a sense of freedom, joy, and inner peace through our conscious, creative choices. This is the very key to creating conscious beginnings. Through our total acceptance and recognition of our impulses as well as the use of our integrated power we can begin all our interactions and creations with full consciousness and clear intentions.

Question: How do you feel about creating more conscious beginnings in your life?

Conscious Endings

With the same intentions we used to create conscious beginnings, we can establish, explore and create our intention for an ending. We can consider how we want our relationship or connection to end. Do we want it to end painfully, sweetly, as friends, or as enemies? These are all options and possibilities as we create our experiences, so why not create endings that we feel good about?

Exercise: Transforming the fear of letting go

This exercise helps us to explore our feelings of letting go of loved ones.

Let's take a moment now to write down our fears and our pain around the ending of our relationships, be it with a friend, lover, or family member. Let's take our time to be as genuine as we can, while remembering to breathe deeply throughout the process. We can choose to invite our friend, partner, or family member to also do the same process. Through sharing our thoughts on the subject we can transform our dark fears of letting go in the light of day.

One of the most difficult things for us as women to do is to leave the person we love even though they continuously have abused us. Many women say, "I love them and they love me". I often ask those women, "What is love? Is it love to degrade, hurt and control another person?" No. It is not. We can love something that is harmful, yes, yet if we can realize that we still can love this person from a distance that will empower us to take the step towards acting in a loving way towards ourselves. Even if our partner's actions are un-loving, at least our own actions towards ourselves can still show the strength of our self-love. Our masculine essence, the part of us that keeps us safe, has not been protecting us and we must let that part of us stand for what we feel is right for us. We do not need to be ashamed of desiring respect and honor. We do not have to be afraid to leave what is not fully supportive of all that we are. We can love ourselves enough to leave.

Exercise: Loving ourselves enough to ensure our own safety

The following exercises are useful for getting clarity on our current situations so we may consciously choose how we wish to live.

At some point in our lives we will be confronted with people and situations that do not support who we truly are despite the fact that we still love these people. Answering this following question is unique for each of us, let's take the time now to answer honestly: "Do you love yourself enough to care for yourself as much or more than those for whom you feel love?"

Knowing that love is not disrespectful, possessive, controlling, fearful and abusive, our natural curiosity of *what love is arises*. Bears Koffman shares a wonderful concept of what love is in his infamous quote, "love is to be happy with". This simple construct enables a person to experience the pleasure of loving without conditions. The Art of Succulent Living encourages us to live with an open heart while being interconnected with others and our environment. As sensual women, we understand love is respectful, accepting, detached, patient, kind and natural, and that it allows others the freedom to be who they truly are. This understanding of love gives us the power to consciously end relationships that are not life-giving.

Exercise: Creating conscious endings

This exercise helps us to leave any connection feeling whole and loving.

Another method that promotes conscious endings is to have the person, which we either want to let go of or have the fear of letting go of, share where they are at mentally and emotionally. We can then reciprocate by sharing our own feelings and thoughts. Once this has happened, we can both give thanks for the time we have had together. In this way, we both can enter a quiet, meditative state wherein we can consciously cut cords from each other.

***Energetic cords** are formed with all our connections. This is especially true for the strong energetic cords formed during sexual encounters as compared to cords formed in friendship and in families. This is due to the nature of sexual energy and its bonding qualities. Thus, clearing these cords requires a conscious effort.*

Let's imagine taking a sharp knife and cutting through the cords between our partner and ourselves. Whichever method we use, intention is really the key. Both parties must consciously intend to take back their energy from the other. This reclaiming of chi returns us to a virginal state.

Dissolving Our Past Connections

If cords from past relationships are not adequately cleared, a few things may occur. Often, when a cord is cut or dissolved over time (a period of seven years has been the typical lifespan of a cord), the person who was corded to us may attempt to re-cord themselves. This can show up in many ways, the most common form being an old lover that shows up after a long period of separation. What can we do in these circumstances? One way to clear old cords is to bring our awareness to their existence and then consciously choose to cut them. Having a person who is familiar with clearing the energy body can also be helpful if we don't know how to let go of something we cannot really sense.

Questions: Have you noticed any old lovers come back into your life after a period of time? What did you choose to do when they showed up?

Exercise: Ceremony of cord cutting

This ceremony is for releasing others and reclaiming our lost energy.

When we are aware of the cords (energy links) between ourselves and another and we wish to clear them, we can take a moment to give thanks for all that person has brought into our life. Then either using a real knife or an imagined one, cut through the cords one by one by visualizing the energetic cords in your mind and seeing the knife slicing through the cords. We can visualize our chi going back into us and imagine the other person receiving their chi back as well. Looking at the roots of the cords, we watch them dissolve completely until nothing is left. Asking that the highest good come to that person, we then run our orbit (see Chapter 7, micro-cosmic orbit) for a few minutes. Then we just relax and breathe deeply. When we sense a return of our energy, we welcome it back through acknowledging its return.

Transforming Our Memories

It is important to understand that memories are not real. In fact, we can actually choose to change a memory into anything we desire. For example, if we had a bad experience with someone and, after many years, we are still holding onto resentment or pain connected to this event, we are actually continuing to give our vital energy to these memories and keeping them intact. So it is indeed healthier for us to cut cords with our memories.

To see the innocence in everyone may at first seem very difficult, but it is actually very freeing. Seeing this innocent quality in the context of our painful experiences transforms our perceptions from fear to love and empowers us towards healing. The more we accept our pain as our guide, showing us where we need to love and accept ourselves more, the more we are filled with gratitude and healing energy. Once we realize that we no longer need the memories of pain to remind us of our capacity for love, we can then begin to let go of our past and the cords of our memories will dissolve effortlessly.

Questions: Are you still holding on to negative feelings about someone or a situation? How is holding on to this pain limiting you or helping you to live more fully and freely?

Practicing the Art of Succulent Living means choosing to live fully in present time. Putting ourselves in other people's shoes and seeing ourselves from their perspective can also be an interesting and enlightening experience. The practices of the inner smile and the six healing sounds (see Chapter 7) are instrumental in reclaiming our innate inner peace and deep sense of love and freedom.

Exercise: Transforming negative emotions

This exercise helps to release our judgments.

Each time we have a negative emotion associated with another person, we first cut cords from that person, and then practice smiling into the parts of us that are in need of love and healing. Generating unconditional love within ourselves through our open heart center allows the chi of unconditional love to spread throughout our body.

Walking consciously through our life requires effort, yet the results are so liberating that mindless activity loses its appeal. The more we can become aware of our intention, the more we will become active in creating the life we want. This brings us more energy and vitality as youthfulness is a state of mind. When we live authentically, honoring both others and ourselves, we free up burdensome energy and feel more vibrant and alive.

Lovers are potent people in our lives. They share with us in deep and intimate ways that we are sometimes completely unaware of. It is important to honor the gifts they bring to us and to remember that we too bring gifts to each person we meet and unite with.

Question: When was the last time you spent time thanking your lover(s) for the roles they have played in your life?

Our past experiences are our gifts to ourselves, and we need to use them as such instead of viewing them as limitations. Let our past gift us with its wisdom of *what not to do*. Whatever we chose to do in the past can be honored in its own right. Whatever we did then, we did to the best of our understanding and abilities. The beauty of life is that every moment presents us with the opportunity to make new choices. We are not confined to patterns. We can choose to act in ways we have never dreamed of before. Whatever we choose, if we are listening carefully, we will know that it is right because our body will let us know. When something is not right we feel insecure, stressed and anxious. When something is right we feel centered, elated and alive.

Question: How do you view your past, as a burden or as a gift?

The only constant in life is not just *change*, but *choice*. Every moment, is an opportunity to exercise our power to choose that which is in the highest interest for all. Every moment we create the life we live. As long as we practice making our choices consciously, choosing our beginnings, endings and everything in between will become easier and easier. When we live our truth and walk the path of bliss, it is very important to have conscious heart-opening beginnings while also being aware of our conscious cord-cutting endings. Most of our problems, issues and memories are partly due to the fact that we have not known what it is to end a relationship (romantic or not) with awareness, clarity and closure.

Questions: Have you ever consciously ended a relationship? How would you want your relationship to end?

Life is a rhythm of beginnings and endings, one flowing into the other in a constant cycle/recycle pattern. Becoming aware of this and knowing how to work with this truth can be very liberating and healing.

Conscious Relationships

There are multiple reasons for choosing to be in a relationship. No reason is right or wrong. It is simply an expression of who we believe ourselves to be in the moment we are making that choice. If the experience of a relationship took away from our life or somehow we felt "less-than", that connection is considered to be life-taking. If, instead, the experience of the relationship enhances our life, the connection would then be life-giving and would lead to both partners realizing more of who they truly are.

But what would happen if our partner's life-giving choice was to have sex with someone other than us? If we view sex as simply a human pleasure, this will help us release fears or negative beliefs around sexuality and to understand that before a person is a partner that they are also naturally a sexual being. So why would being in relationship create a fear in us?

> Question: Is sex with your partner an unconscious, life-taking choice or a conscious life-giving choice?

The life-giving choice in a relationship would be the conscious choice *to never limit* a partner and to support that person to experience life as fully as possible by empowering their life-giving choices. When we freely allow ourselves to choose pleasure through eating a juicy peach, swimming in the ocean, meditating on a gorgeous landscape, or simply breathing, we will find an increase in our desire for allowing others the same freedom of choice. This can equally be applied to sexual choices. The Art of Succulent Living allows freedom for everyone to choose their version of sexual pleasure, including their choice of sexual partners.

> Questions: Why are you or are you not in relationship? Do you believe that you are responsible for your partner's happiness or pleasure? Do you feel drawn to define what your partner should or should not do with their life, especially their sexual choices?

Once we free our partners and ourselves to make sexual choices, we begin to understand sex as being one of the body's many ways of experiencing pleasure. Remembering that orgasm can occur independently of sex, why would we choose to connect sexually? If sex is enacted due to boredom, obligation, exhaustion, stress, or any other circumstance inhibiting full presence, it becomes merely an act of releasing internal tension. Sex when horny is not necessary (though plenty of fun). Also, sex for the sake of rekindling intimacy (which has often diminished due to the unwillingness to open our heart) is also not necessary (though also plenty of fun). These are life-taking forms of sexual expression.

> Questions: What kind of sexual exchanges have you experienced: life-giving or life-taking? If you were to choose now, which kind of sexual connection would you prefer? How would you turn a life-taking connection into a life-giving connection?

If we redefine sexual exchange as being a sacred communion between two conscious beings, then the reason for sex becomes one of celebration, an expression of life-giving sexuality. Communion in celebration of sexuality is only possible when our mind-body-soul is present and available to participate fully with another totally present person. Imagine that sex is the result of two (or more) energies coming together in conscious, alive openness. This sacred union occurs not only through the genitals but also through the emotions/heart, the mind, and the spirit. This is the vibration of succulent sex.

Celebrating the Power of Choice

In the old fear-based paradigm, it is common to witness people make promises based on their fears, be it a fear of being abandoned, being alone, being betrayed, or being just like everyone else. Choosing a partner while feeling obliged, pressured or comfortable and safe in the routine of the relationship is not an expression of love, but rather of fear.

The new paradigm of the Art of Succulent Living weaves the experience of bliss and joy into each and every precious moment, independent of any external influences. As sensual women, we view external things as simply there for sharing in our pure joy of celebration. We regard life as sacred and view every act of life as precious and equal. Living as sensual women we exercise our freedom to make life-giving choices. The love-based choices of allowing freedom, honesty, openness, authenticity and the genuine desire to see the other be all they can be permeates all of our relationships. When we honor these life-giving choices in our partner and ourselves, we are participating in the ultimate expression of love: being together by conscious choice. The highest expression of love is exercising our freedom of choice and using our power to consciously create from this integrated place.

"A common liability of fear is that it inhibits our ability to be present and our ability to take care of ourselves."

— BEARS KOFFMAN

CHAPTER QUESTIONS

How does the idea of conscious living and creating conscious beginnings, endings, and choices feel to you and is it something you will implement into your life?

Through understanding the different energies of love, lust and procreative urges, how will this influence your sexual choices?

Exploring the art of succulent living exposes the idea of creating from fear/limitation or from love/conscious choice. How does this knowledge affect your view of life and sexuality?

CHAPTER FIVE

From Multi-Orgasm to Omni-Orgasm

Expanding Our Understanding
of the Orgasmic Experience

I am a tender blossom
of exotic
proportions

petals extended

open, willing, ready

to receive
the warm penetrative
force
of the Father Sun
and
the nurturing coolness
of the Mother Earth

I need nothing else

as simply
being
is an act
of the most
profound

Ecstasy

LIVING WITH DEEP CONSCIOUS AWARENESS of all our impulses involves activating our innate wisdom to make life-giving choices, especially when it comes to our sexuality. When we merge the heightened awareness of our mind with the expanded sensuality of our body, we begin to access a realm of virtually limitless pleasure. If we are to expand our concept of orgasm to include the multiple orgasm and the omni-orgasm, we must first redefine what an orgasm is, then redefine ourselves as sensual women as we access greater understanding and mastery of our own orgasmic energy.

What is Orgasm?

Orgasm: the infamous word invoking a range of responses from desire, longing and frustration to awe-inspiring, life-enhancing bliss. Most women feel they have never had an orgasm or are unsure if they have even experienced anything close to one. The word orgasm stems from the Greek word *orgainein* which means "to engorge with lust". As sensual women, if we want to cultivate a healthy understanding of what an orgasm is, we must investigate how the seemingly ordinary definition of "engorging with lust" could lead to the bone-shaking, mind-altering moments of ecstasy that embody the actual experience of orgasm.

> ORGASM: The climax of coitus, consisting of a series of involuntary muscle contractions in the anus, lower pelvic muscles, and sexual organs, accompanied by a sudden release of endorphins providing a feeling of euphoria.

This definition defines orgasm as simply being *coitus*, the sexual union of a man and a woman, but it leaves out the orgasmic sensations created by self-pleasuring and by same-sex coupling. It also limits orgasm to intercourse. Not all of us engage in sexual intercourse with men, and of those of us who do, few of us attain orgasm through penetration. So does this mean that many of us are not experiencing orgasm at all?

Restricting ourselves to such a limited definition of orgasm limits our understanding and, thus, our actual experience of it. The Jade Goddess teachings moves beyond this limited understanding to explore many other ways of accessing this powerful orgasmic chi. In order to develop our mastery of this powerful energy, we must embrace a new, expanded definition of orgasm.

Questions: What is your current definition of orgasm? With this definition, would you say you experience orgasm or not?

When I was a teenager I was very sexual with myself. I had my first release of ambrosia (ejaculation) when I was twelve years old (after starting my period) and had many very expanded and pleasurable sexual experiences as a result. At that time, I was very curious about the adult's whispers on orgasm. "What was it? Did I experience it?" From the definitions I found in dictionaries and encyclopedias, I concluded that I did not have orgasms. In fact, no information I ever found on the subject included a description of the sensations of intense pleasure and the high I would get on my own. Years later as an adult, after speaking to men and women about the subject of orgasm, I realized that I had indeed experienced orgasm and had done so for as long as I could remember. It was so funny the first time a lover asked me, "So, did you cum?", and I replied, "I have no idea." Now I know that I have had many blissful orgasms and that there is nothing wrong with me.

Questions: What is your earliest memory of orgasm? Is it easy for you to orgasm? Or do you feel you have never had one?

It is valuable for all women, especially young adults, to have access to accurate information that can empower our sexuality and satiate our curiosities. When we share our stories, we realize that we are not alone and that, as highly sensual beings, we are perfectly natural. Keeping this in mind, let's look at another definition of orgasm:

> An orgasm, also known as a climax, is a pleasurable physiological, and to no small degree a psychological, response to sexual stimulation that can be experienced by both males and females. Orgasm is the third stage of four in the human sexual response cycle, the currently accepted model of the physiological process of sexual stimulation. It is the conclusion of the plateau phase in a release of sexual tension. Both males and females experience quick cycles of muscle contraction of the anus and lower pelvic muscles, as well as in the sexual organs.
>
> Orgasms in both men and women are often associated with other involuntary actions, including vocalizations and muscular spasms in other areas of the body. Also, a generally euphoric sensation is associated with orgasm. Orgasm generally causes perceived tiredness, and both males and females often feel a need to rest afterwards. This is often attributed to the release of endorphins during orgasm causing relaxation and drowsiness, but can also be due to the body's need for a short rest after a bout of vigorous sexual activity.

This formal description not only limits the experience of orgasm to the physiological—pelvic muscles, hormones, etc.—it also states the commonly accepted myth that humans by nature become tired from sex. However, according to

Taoist sexology, if we do not know how to redirect our orgasmic energy and circulate it, it is wasted; thus, we become depleted or tired. But when we learn how to redirect the orgasmic chi through the micro-cosmic orbit and into the organs, glands and bones, we become very energized and revitalized from sex.

The encyclopedia also describes orgasm as being a vigorous activity. But this leaves out all the subtle expressions of sexual excitement. Ancient Taoists developed many ways of staying completely relaxed, alert and aroused for many, many hours. In fact, sometimes the techniques are so subtle, it looks like the practitioner is sleeping! What is exciting about all of this, is that there is so much more to tap into when it comes to sex and orgasm.

As sensual women seeking to redefine our understanding of orgasm, we must open our minds and bodies to accept the possibility of experiencing what we have never known was possible, while keeping an objective perspective of what is possible. Many of us have had orgasmic experiences, yet we have either devalued them or disbelieved them because we did not have any previous knowledge or understanding of what it was we were experiencing. These non-defined orgasmic experiences feel very real and juicy. They are delightful and inexplicable. Instead of overlooking them, why not embrace them? My desire to redefine orgasm comes from having direct experiences of what has not been previously explained. Will we automatically choose to ignore very real body experiences due to a lack of acceptable definitions, or will we choose to trust our body's innate wisdom?

Questions: Have you ever experienced a non-genital orgasm? Can you recall any time in your life where you may have experienced ecstatic pleasure in your body?

The Pursuit of Orgasm

Why do we innately seem to yearn for the experience of orgasm? Even those who have renounced sex still seek orgasm, the feeling of total oneness with whatever it is they most desire, be it God, the Earth, a person, or any other object of desire. In investigating the reasons for the pull to orgasm, we must look at the context in which it occurs. Orgasm only happens in present time. It doesn't exist in the past or future. It is only experienced in this moment, not yesterday or tomorrow. Thus, orgasm is a way that humans seek to be fully in the *now*. The now is without past or future, it is when we are so absorbed by the experience of the moment we are in, that we completely forget about our past and future. When we are present in this way, even just for a few seconds, we feel more alive, blissful and free.

The Energetic Map of Orgasm

While many things occur in the moment of orgasm, one of the most important aspects is that within the instant of orgasm, there is a sense of being at one with ourselves. All our energy is activated and we have access to our inner truth, the Divine within. Whether we believe we can access the Divine or not, it still happens. Today, many of us have lost our sense of self, our centers, and the presence of the Divine and sacred in our lives. We seek orgasm as a way to reconnect to our **Source**. Our seeking is often unconscious since we do not always know what motivates us to naturally yearn for orgasm. Many of us say it is because "it feels good" or that it makes us "relax". But many things feel good and help us relax, yet are not as desirable as orgasm. Why?

Orgasm is the ultimate moment. Even those of us who have never had one still pursue it with some understanding that it is an experience we must have at least once in our life. For those of us who question the relationship of the sacred and Divine to sex and especially to orgasm, we may want to try redefining sex as an act of sacred communion.

Questions: What is your personal understanding of orgasm and spirituality? Do you view sex as something profane or sinful or do you see it as a sacred act?

When we lack understanding about our sexual chi, we restrict ourselves to a short-lived, genitally focused normal orgasm. When we expand our mind and body to understand genital orgasm as merely the starting point, then a world of infinite possibilities opens to us. The more our entire body, mind and heart are involved in experiencing the orgasm, the bigger and longer and more intense it becomes. This can be compared to any sensual experience—if we just involve one of our senses the experience is ok; but if we involve *all* of our senses, then the same experience comes alive, rich with sensuality.

Orgasm is our *birthright*. The more we have them, the more alive we become. This refers to multiple orgasms for both men (without seminal release) and women (possibly with release). Orgasm is our doorway to bliss. It is not the end point, but the entry point to a whole new dimension of living. The more aroused we are, the more vibrant we become. The more we allow life to touch us in ways that invoke orgasm, the more rich and full our lives become. We will no longer pursue happiness outside of ourselves—instead, it will become something that is innate within us, released and cultivated through our ecstatic response to life.

The Multi-Orgasm or Multiple Orgasm

Now that we have looked at the concept of orgasm and seen both its limited definitions and its potential, we are now ready to look at the infamous multiple orgasm or multi-orgasm. The multiple orgasm has been the subject of many books and discussions over the last decade. While this phenomenon is often commonly associated with (and sometimes believed to be restricted to) the feminine expression of sexual experience, research shows that the masculine expression of sexual activation is also multi-orgasmic.

Multi means many, thus *multi-orgasm* is the ability to have many orgasms within the context of one sexual encounter. This may occur many times within one moment or many times in successive moments. The act of having multi-orgasms is potentially available to all of us if we choose to learn to access this ability and work on cultivating this experience.

> *Questions: What has your understanding been of a multi-orgasm? Have you ever experienced one?*

Omni-Orgasm

Omni-orgasm is a term I developed many years ago to define my own personal sexual orientation. The birth of the omni-orgasm came with both the realization that *life* itself is arousing and with my refusal to be defined by or limited to the usual categories used to describe sexual orientation: heterosexual, homosexual, bisexual, transsexual or gender-fluid. All these labels assume that our potential for sexual experience is reserved to that of human interaction. Sadly, this leaves out the rest of life.

The term omni-orgasm means all-orgasmic. This is an important definition of orgasm as it expands sexual potential beyond the constraints of our modern-day definition. Omni-orgasmic implies that our whole body is orgasmic, thus removing the responsibility of orgasm from our genitals and expanding it to every cell in our body. True orgasm occurs in the **master glands** of the brain, where endorphins are released to create the euphoric high of orgasm. But we also have the potential to send orgasmic sensation to literally any part of our body at will. This gives us a much broader canvas on which to paint our erotic experiences.

All of life is rich with orgasmic potential. Being omni-orgasmic women means embracing a greater understanding of our senses and our inherent capacity to receive and experience pleasure. In this state, we could find a sunset so beautiful that it literally excites the pleasure sensors of our brain into a full body orgasm. Our whole human experience (life) contains within it the limitless possibility for omni-orgasmic bliss. We can free ourselves from the burden of being the sole providers of ecstasy when we embrace the concept that life itself is ecstasy.

Finally, omni-orgasm has the potential to evolve into something greater than what anyone has imagined. It has a component of the Divine within it. For some of us, the concept of uniting spirituality and sexuality may seem a bit far-fetched, but by opening up our critical minds, we can make room for limitless possibilities. As soon as we define *something*—how things can or cannot be—we are unable to access its potential.

Questions: How does this information on omni-orgasm make you feel? In what way would you redefine this explanation to fit into your reality?

Moving from Multi-Orgasm to Omni-Orgasm

At every moment, our body is performing an incredible act of creation. The DNA of our cells is in constant and fluid motion, making love and creating new life over and over again. With such a rich resource of energy in our body—up to a hundred trillion cells—it is a wonder why any of us are unhappy and dissatisfied. A large part of the Taoist teachings are based on activating formulas that train our mind to sense this deeper phenomenon of our body—the constant ecstasy of our replicating cells. If we are aware of our body and are able to open, clean and clear, we will be able to receive and perceive all the subtle yet orgasmic messages of our body. The more we can access this inner world, the deeper our understanding and mastery of the subtle patterns of ecstasy will be.

Omni-orgasm is a new way of understanding and defining orgasm. It is the *message* or *signal* sent throughout every cell of our body. It is our *aliveness*. When we tune into the subtle yet incredible sensation of our trillions of cells shimmering or pulsing, we connect with our full body or omni-orgasmic state. The Jade Goddess teachings enable us to become familiar and comfortable with our entire body as a sensual vessel of bliss.

We could still have an omni-orgasmic experience that is initially felt in the genitals, but we would no longer have to limit our sources of stimulation to those that are typically sexual. For example, we may experience our bliss simply by eating a delicious meal or indulging in a rich aroma.

The more we can surrender to the fullness of the moment, the more receptive we become to the subtle movement of pleasure throughout our whole body, mind and spirit. Some of my students have gone from never having experienced an orgasm (in the traditional sense) to experiencing intense full-body omni-orgasms. This is not accomplished by willing it, but by being fully present with whatever is.

Question: Would you be willing to believe you are a pleasure-full being?

Omni-Orgasm in Everyday Life

Every moment we live is precious. By accessing the ability to live fully in each moment, we become whole. Living in the present—in the now—we experience our totality, our omni-orgasmic state. We can practice sharing this bliss in every aspect of our life. How magnificent! How is this done? Though often seen as impossible, it is rather simple: all that is needed is to surrender fully to the beauty of the moment no matter what we are experiencing.

Exercise: Expanding into an omni-orgasmic state

We can practice breathing deeply and allowing our whole body to drink in the life that surrounds us. As we taste something, it is *all* of us tasting. If we see something beautiful, it is *all* of us seeing. If we smell something, it is *all* of us allowing the scent to fully penetrate us. Through doing this with all of our senses we access the present moment fully.

The more we practice being fully present, the more we access this new way of walking through life. The boring sparkles, the normal becomes supernatural; the plain or unseen becomes spectacular. What has changed? The external? No, we have changed from the inside out. The more we give ourselves permission to experience the innate ecstasy that exists within us, the more we experience it on the outside. As sensual women, we allow life to gift itself to us. We make room within ourselves to fully surrender, not to an event or person or thing, but to life itself and what inherently imbues it. We surrender to the love that impregnates everything.

Exercise: Celebrating all of life

When a beautiful person stands near us, rather then comparing ourselves and then putting them or ourselves down, let's drink in their beauty. To acknowledge another person's beauty, talent, success, etc., allows us to celebrate with them. Through this celebration, we expand and become more open and vibrant, as do they. Recognizing the vibrant life force within people, we acknowledge the same vibrancy living inside of us. This is where the saying, "we are all one", comes in. We can celebrate everyone, including ourselves through saying inwardly, "I celebrate all that you are. Thank you for being in my life now".

Questions: Does the idea of becoming aware of every sensual experience resonate with you? Is it possible for you to celebrate the people in your life?

In the world of separation, we make the things that we fear wrong and the things we desire right. In the world of omni-orgasm, we embrace everything and see it all as an act of love. On the subtlest levels of physical life, the subatomic levels of our existence, the positive and negative (yang and yin), are dancing. All of life has this movement, even inanimate objects. In the world of omni-orgasm, we become much bigger, more available to the wonder and glory of what it is to truly be alive. As sensual women, we do not just reserve this for special occasions, but we always live from this place.

As we live from this place, we begin to feel that it is normal to be blissful, and unusual to be in fear or misery. This does not mean that we never experience hurt or react with anger, sadness or fear. In fact, we will continue to have these rich human experiences until the day we choose a new journey: death. The difference with omni-orgasmic living is that even if we feel the pain of loss, the heat of anger, or the paralysis of fear, we sense that we are alive. We allow ourselves to feel, and we use these feelings to guide us to transform our negative experiences into powerful, rejuvenating energy.

Questions: What is your normal state of being? Do you believe that life has to be hard? Do you see life as an opportunity to shine your radiance?

Being Fully Present and Open to the Omni-Orgasmic State

The first step to realizing omni-orgasmic states of living is being willing to accept that being omni-orgasmic is both realistic and possible. Next, we must focus on our *self* as the subject of cultivation, versus using a video, toy, person or situation. Finally, when we experience an orgasm, instead of holding our breath (a common instinctual reaction), we practice breathing very slowly and deeply, allowing our breath to move into our whole body, and we feel as though our every cell is receiving the orgasmic charge. Our full participation in all things is the key to omni-orgasmic, succulent living.

Pain and Beyond

Pain is the other side of our ecstasy, which is probably why the **BDSM (Bondage S&M)** culture is growing rapidly. There is so much pain in the world and people have found a way to use pain to push them into the other side: pleasure. But, numbing any part of ourselves limits our potential for experiencing bliss. Habitual sexual patterns such as "getting off" create **dead zones** in us, parts of us that have stopped being present to our aliveness. Instead of creating more dead zones and numbness through our experiences of pain, we can awaken and revitalize these zones by becoming fully present and aware of our life force.

Omni-orgasmic living, unlike normal orgasmic experience, does not require any external stimulation. In fact, when first training our body to remember omni-orgasm, it is best not to use too much stimulation or external sources of pleasure. When we are patterned to use external methods, we can re-pattern ourselves by increasing our sensitivity through turning our attention inwards and expanding the sensation of bliss throughout our body.

Exercise: Increasing our orgasmic experience in daily life

The next time we are in a situation that is pleasurable (but not orgasmic), simply recall the feeling of orgasm. Allow it to fill us fully in this moment. Through our awareness we allow ourselves to induce the sensation of orgasm and let it spread through our whole body while relaxing and breathing slowly. Smiling and having a playful attitude while making pleasurable sounds can also help.

Question: Do you believe that an external factor such as a partner, sex toys, sex videos, romantic settings, drugs, or alcohol is responsible for your pleasure?

Our Omni-Orgasmic Potential

For some of us who have deeply ingrained sexual habits, the thought of having multiple or omni-orgasms and transforming our dead zones into greater aliveness and bliss may seem like too much work. As sensual women, however, it is not work but the simple choice of changing our limited attitudes into unlimited choices. We transform our separation into wholeness as our need for external stimulus relaxes and is replaced by our own unique way of accessing the wealth of our internal bliss.

"Ananda – bliss consciousness (Sanskrit meaning the ecstasy of love), whatever brings you closer to wholeness, brings you closer to ecstasy"

– DEEPAK CHOPRA

The truth is we were created by orgasm. Two sex cells merged to become one whole. From this orgasmic union of yin and yang (egg and sperm), our whole being came to be. In fact, every cell that is created from that point still comes from the dividing of this original union. Therefore, each cell in our body is inundated with the energy of orgasmic creation.

Bliss is our birthright. The only thing holding us back from experiencing omni-orgasm is our own belief. Our inherited beliefs have led us to falsely believe that we are not beings of *bliss*. This is a crime. These limiting beliefs have created a world of people who fear their own creative (sexual) power. At any moment this can change, for limiting beliefs are creations of our mind and we can transmute them into new, empowering beliefs. Our ability to shape our lives through what we choose to believe and think is the key to accessing our full conscious awareness of ourselves. How we choose to define ourselves with this understanding is a unique and creative journey.

Exercise: Choosing new, empowering beliefs

Let's take a moment to write down our thoughts, ideas, beliefs and concepts that we sense may no longer support who we know ourselves to be: a beautiful, radiant, blissful being. Now, for each belief, state the following: I release the belief _____ (old limiting belief). I now choose to believe _____ (new expansive belief).

It's helpful for us to repeat our new choices regularly, particularly whenever we hear our old beliefs acting out. Through smiling radiant love into our heart and letting it spread throughout our body, we open ourselves to recreating our reality in our own unique way.

Accepting our orgasmic potential to include both multi-orgasms and omni-orgasms, we are able to stretch beyond the limited definitions of our bliss. Through this gracious acceptance of our pleasure we empower ourselves to transform our sensual/sexual relationship with both others and ourselves.

CHAPTER QUESTIONS

How does understanding "orgasm as your birthright" lead to your exploration of living a succulent life?

Are you ready to explore the possibility that everything you experience in life is your own creation, and that you have the power to expand or change it?

CHAPTER SIX

Shiva and Shakti

The Dance of the Divine Masculine
and the Divine Feminine

Shiva
charmed you have me
full of delightful
bursts of bubbling bliss

though many have
come to sample the
exotic flavor of this garden
none have been gifted
the nectar

this is reserved for you, oh Shiva

for I long for your lips
to taste my honey succulence
and through this intoxication
of Divine beauty
we shall dance
beneath the silky sky
forgetting that time exists

the priceless gift of
passions' enchantment

As sensual women practicing the Art of Succulent Living, we have expanded our orgasmic consciousness by harnessing our innate bliss and by realizing this bliss is essentially our sole creation. Knowing that we create our own orgasmic experiences, we now bring our attention to the role of men in our lives. According to the Taoist understanding of yin and yang energies, the gift of masculine energy is that it harmonizes and heals our own feminine energy as we emerge more fully as sensual women.

Men! Shivas!

Shiva and *Shakti* are Sanskrit words used in the Vedic teachings of ancient India to describe the male and female energies of the cosmos. Shiva represents the Masculine as found in men, solar energy, and cosmic consciousness or awareness, while Shakti represents the Feminine as found in women, lunar energy, and cosmic energy. This Vedic concept is harmonious with the ancient Taoist cosmology of polar opposites found in yin-yang, soft-hard, negative-positive, and female-male. In our daily life, we find the manifestation of Shiva, the Divine Masculine energy, in our relations with our brothers, fathers, lovers, husbands, sons and friends, and within ourselves.

As women, the ambassadors of Shakti, the Divine Feminine, we dis-empower ourselves when we claim not to understand men and claim to be frustrated, hurt, abused and imprisoned by them. If we were to truly own our own power and be at peace with our own masculine energy, would we still feel such things? A common statement about our masculine counterparts such as "we can't live without them, we can't live with them", separates us from the Masculine. In truth, we all are both yin-yang, female-male. Once we bring this understanding into our compassion practice (harmonizing our yin/sexual energy with our yang/heart energy), we find that we attain greater peace and joy in all our relations with men. Transforming our on-off relationship with men and the Masculine into our own inner and outer masculine energies, we personally benefit by feeling more balanced and whole.

Another common belief that limits the potential of male and female relationships is found when a man enters a relationship hoping that a woman will never change, yet to his disappointment, she does; or when a woman enters a relationship hoping that a man will change, and to her disappointment, he doesn't. When these situations occur, both partners have forgotten to celebrate the unique essence of a man and woman, not in personality, but in energy, in the expression of the Divine Masculine/Shiva and the Divine Feminine/Shakti.

Question: What is the role of men in your life?

The Art of Succulent Living requires the understanding of the interconnection of the male and female energies. If we look closely at the Taoist theory of yin and yang energy patterns, we begin to see their existence within men and women, and more profoundly understand life's dynamics and our relationship patterns. In general, we can define women as yin in nature: receptive, mysterious, watery, able to house life. Conversely, we can define men as yang in nature: penetrative, protective, fiery, able to provide for life.

When we embrace our own Masculine energy, we empower ourselves to make choices out of love and not fear. We often fear what we do not understand. The more we get to know our own yang, the more we will be open to the yang of others. As sensual women, we must also realize that when it comes to men, more compassion is the key to a harmonious connection. Men have challenges just as we do, and it is a misconception to believe otherwise.

Question: What is your present understanding of men and their energy, be it sexual and otherwise?

In some respects, our brothers (men) have a harder time than we do. For one, they do not have the freedom to express their emotions. This alone can cause severe imbalances in the body. Furthermore, they do not have the same capabilities to internally reference themselves as women do. For example, consider the location of their genitals. Located outside of their body, the male genitals give men the ability to externally reference their sexuality, whereas we women have our genitals neatly tucked away, forcing us to develop an internal awareness of our sexuality. Thus, just from looking at the differences in the placement of our genitals, we can see how we as women develop a keener sense of the inner body, whereas men develop a keener sense of the external body. The Taoists also see the general energy pattern for yin as being internal and yang as being external.

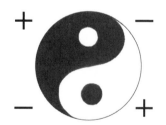

Fig. 6.1 Dynamics of Yin and Yang
How energy moves through women and men

Another vital energetic concept that is very important to understand lies in how men and women interact with the world around them. Men and women penetrate the world in different ways. Our breasts, external expression of our heart, are what we penetrate the world with; whereas a man penetrates the world with his vajra (penis), the external expression of his sexuality. In harmony with their penetrative energies, men and women receive the world in different ways. We women receive the world through our yoni (vulva), whereas a man receives it through his chest/heart.

This key dynamic impacts how succulent, conscious women choose to interact with men. The feminine heart is the +/yang expression, the energy with which women penetrate men. If this heart penetration is done forcefully (such as when we say "tell me your feelings"), a form of emotional rape or emotional invasion may occur. The reverse is true for men if they penetrate a woman with their +/yang pole (vajra). When this penetration is unwanted, it is considered sexual rape or sexual invasion.

Questions: Have you ever attempted to find out how a man is feeling? Or judged his feelings or lack of connection to his feelings?

It is equally important to understand how our desires and our needs as women to be met and seen for who we really are—as Shakti, the Divine Feminine—are actually reciprocated in men. Men also want to be honored as Shiva, the Divine Masculine, to have their inner desires seen and met. Generally, people want to be loved and accepted unconditionally as they are. The difference lies in how men and women choose to express this desire. As women, we expect to be met emotionally—this is where we are comfortable, as it is our outward/yang form of expression. On the other hand, men expect to be met sexually—this is where they are comfortable, as it is their outward/yang form of expression.

The key to overcoming this imbalance lies in honoring the yin/feminine expression of both sexes. For women, that means honoring our yoni, while for men, that means honoring their heart. We can see by this example how women and men penetrate the world. There are few times in modern society where a woman's yoni is approached tenderly, gently and with reverence, and where a man's heart is approached with gentleness, understanding and respect. As sensual women, we are wise to recognize this imbalance and encourage the reunion of our own Masculine with our Feminine, our heart with our yoni.

Historically, both men and women have played imbalanced roles. Women were seen as male property existing solely to propagate the family or male seed. Our yin pole, our yoni, was not considered a sacred place, but a place to satisfy a man's desire and to bear the fruit of his loins, while our positive pole, our heart, characterized us as being devoted, loving and emotional beings. On the same note, men's yin pole (his heart) was not cultivated. His warlike nature, his ability to do and conquer was a higher priority. A man was considered a sissy or worse if he allowed his emotions to surface let alone guide him. Rape was considered a normal male activity. This unbalanced cultivation of men's and women's energies birthed many of the social issues we now face today.

The return to harmony is a natural part of the Universe's mysterious balancing act. Today, people are faced with new options—new ways of thinking, acting and being. As more and more men and women recognize their own inherent value and the value of harmonizing the energy within themselves, they will begin to seek the same externally in others. This desire for cultivating harmony and seeking balance is a hallmark of those of us who practice the Art of Succulent Living.

> *Questions: What is the value of recognizing this concept of yin and yang poles in men and women? What steps can you take to observe this phenomenon, and begin the journey to cultivating harmony?*

Honoring a Man's Yin Expression

When a man opens his heart, lives from his heart, or even simply feels from his heart, he feels vulnerable. This is due to the yin expression of this part of his make-up. A man needs to explore this aspect of himself and realize on his own that being yin (soft, receptive) does not in any way diminish his yang (male energy), but rather, enhances it. The more a man comes into contact with his yin and nurtures it, the more freedom he will give his yang. Typically, being a "real man" means "not crying, taking punches, and doing what it takes even if it hurts". But being a real man cannot be attained if only this one aspect of him is cultivated. The yin/feminine aspect of a man deepens a man. It allows him to access his intuition, inner wisdom and presence, qualities which enhance the fullness and power of the Divine Masculine essence that lives within him.

When a man is confident enough that he does not need to boast, fight or prove himself, he already knows inside himself that he is already the best he can be at this time. Thus, he becomes free—free to truly just be. It is this art of be-ing or his Shiva presence that makes a man extremely attractive to the Shakti presence within a woman. An example of this is when we women are drawn to taken men. We feel more comfortable and relaxed to be ourselves with these men, even before we know they are married or partnered. Why? These taken men are relaxed and do not need anything from us, but instead they can just be with us. This quality is sexy and attractive.

> *Questions: Have you ever been attracted to men who have a beloved? What did their energy feel like to you? What was attractive about this energy?*

The depth of presence in a man will determine his true attractiveness, not how fit or wealthy he is. Why? Shiva presence holds space for Shakti, our Divine Feminine, to emerge and show herself. She will not show herself if she does not trust the environment. As women, we want to know that we can be all that we are: raging, crying, laughing, moaning and screaming in ecstasy, without fear of being abandoned. We need to trust that our man can handle all of our power, no matter what form it takes.

Women are like water—changing, deep and succulent. Like water, we can express ourselves in many forms, be it snow, hail, rain, mist, or steam. We are an ocean wave crashing against a mountain, all the while trusting that the mountain will be there. Men with presence are like the mountain—strong, still, and present. When we trust this masculine presence, our emotional expression is free to flow through us into stillness. A man's presence not only heals trust in the Masculine, it invites the Feminine to equally hold space for the full range of masculine expression.

Women who do not yet know themselves tend to choose compromising situations that make them feel repressed or shut down. Sensual women, on the other hand, know themselves. They are not afraid to be who they are. As sensual women, we consciously create situations where we can have freedom of expression. Men who do not yet know themselves may unconsciously choose women who resemble their mother, women who are afraid of them or their potential, or women who do not want them to grow up. On the other hand, men who have realized themselves choose women who will love and support them and draw out their potential.

Questions: What sort of relationship do you have with men? Do you see them as your equal or as greater or lesser than you?

Relating from a State of Wholeness

As women practicing the Art of Succulent Living, we seek and express refined levels of relating. We invest solely in enabling others to fully realize their potential. In succulent, conscious relationships, both partners are invested in truth, integrity, love and open, clear communication. They support their partner without holding them back. Cultivating acceptance creates an open-hearted space in which both individuals are free to choose their life experiences without fear of judgment or repression. In these harmonious relationships, be they intimate or friendly, one is able to celebrate the blossoming of each individual. Relating in this way eliminates our fears of abandonment as we realize that we are never alone. The partnership between two *whole* beings is not a vacuum to be filled solely by the other. It is a coming together to share that wholeness. This level of relationship is potentially available to all of us, and it begins in the cultivation of ourselves.

Through the use of the Jade Goddess teachings, the Art of Succulent Living focuses on the attainment of our *wholeness* and of sharing from the space of abundance. As sensual women we literally magnetize to us what and who we are. We draw to us people who are innately equal. No one is more or less than us. That is why as we grow, we may find ourselves seeking new friends and partners unless our friends and partners grow with us. This can be a beautiful thing instead of a frightening thing. When we choose to be what it is we desire in others, we become the love we have always wanted.

> *Questions: How does practicing the Art of Succulent Living through becoming whole unto yourself feel? How does this change your perception of relationship? How would the role of men change in your life?*

The Differences in Male and Female Sexuality

Just as the yin and yang poles express themselves in different ways for men and women, their sexual energy patterns differ. In general, the yin pattern (women) moves from the outside in, whereas the yang pattern (men) moves from the inside out. As women, we prefer the rest of our body to be touched and acknowledged *before* our yoni is given attention. Men on the other hand enjoy having the energy *begin* with their vajra (penis) and then slowly expanded to the rest of their body. This pattern also shows up in the Feminine yearning to be *filled* and the Masculine yearning to be *emptied*. Men and women innately seek what will naturally harmonize and balance them.

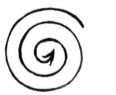

Fig. 6.2 Movement of energy within women (left) and men (right)

To fully activate a woman sexually, we begin with her extremities and slowly work inwards towards her yoni (vulva). There are exceptions to this guideline, yet in general, a woman's energy patterns and body will respond favorably to soft kisses, caresses, massage and attention given to her entire body prior to sexual contact. To fully activate a man, we begin with his vajra (penis) and work outward from there, spreading sexual energy across his whole body with massage, kisses and loving attention, moving from his genitals to the rest of his body. This difference in the feminine and masculine energy flow is often a cause of disharmony in sexual relationships where the woman is rarely ever fully aroused enough to experience total fullness, and where the man is rarely ever fully opened enough to experience total emptiness, the deep stillness of the Universe.

Shiva with Shakti: Exchanging Love

As sensual women loving a man, it is important for us to remember to activate not only our heart, but also our throat and sex centers. Our heart is the midpoint between these two wonderful creative vortexes. Taking responsibility for our own orgasm is part of being a sensual woman—when we do this, we take all the pressure off of our partners. We must also remember to exercise our voice, to speak up when we have sexual desires. This can occasionally be difficult when we feel the fragility of our partners' ego. Sharing the truth about our desires is not about making him wrong or bad. It is about making clear, true, loving requests. In fact, it is sexy for us to say what turns us on, just as it is sexy for a man to relax into hearing and accepting whatever mood we may be in. Our mystery is sexy. Just when men think they have us figured out, they realize that they are nowhere near to understanding our desires.

Exercise: Giving our desire a voice

Speaking of our sexual needs often frighten us. But doing so reveals to us the type of relationship we have. If we choose to share, let's do it from our heart, using the language of "I" instead of "you". Here is an example of a non-heart statement: "You have no idea how to touch my yoni, and if you would only try this or that, it would be much better." Instead, use a heart statement: "When I feel your finger barely touch me, it turns me on so much. I love it when you tease me and make me wait for your tongue". Let's have fun practicing new ways to share our desire with our lovers.

The Ego in Sex: The Need to be Right
versus the Acceptance of Being Open

Having taught many men, I have come to realize that ego plays a critical role in sabotaging their growth. For women, it is the emotions that sabotage our growth. When handling the fragile ego of men, it is important for us to understand that they are not their ego—they are their Divine (Shiva) selves. The ego is only meant as a tool, not as an identity.

A man's ego is not right or wrong, good or bad. Ego serves to identify what has come to pass. For example, a man has sex with a woman for the first time and, in that time, learns certain things about his skill as a lover through the many responses she offers him. If her responses seem positive, he will tell himself to remember what he did so that he can *wow* the next woman he encounters. This logic, however, is fundamentally flawed, as a new lover may not respond like the other woman. But since the man is convinced he has the *right* technique, he forgets to listen and pay attention to the signals his new lover gives him. When she gives him a less than positive response, he is angered or embarrassed as his need to be right, to be *the best she's ever had*, overrides his willingness to accept the gift that she is offering him, the gift of being fully present in the moment and surrendering to the unknown. The unknown is actually the domain of the Feminine: yin energy. It is rich, fertile and uncharted territory, accessible only through trusting our innate intuition and instinct. How can we, as sensual women, gently invite our male partners to step beyond the limitations of *knowing* into the fertile possibilities of the *unknown*?

Ego keeps us in the past and also projecting into the future. The ego's investment in *being something* prohibits us from being receptive to the mystery of the present moment. If men understand that their potency lies not in the knowledge they have collected, but in their presence—their ability to be fully present in the moment—they will win access to their greater potential. This potential affects not only sexuality, but all facets of life.

Knowing this, we as sensual women can speak to the Divine Masculine presence in our male partners and invite their inner power to activate through our open, compassionate hearts. Our lovers truly do desire to please us. They may just not know how. Many men would not want to admit they do not know how, and would rather pretend that they do know how, rather than appear as inexperienced. They would like us to think of them as our most incredible lover ever. For both men and women, being an incredible lover is really more of a matter of having incredible listening skills.

Exercise: Transforming our throat centers

Scenerio: We are being pleasured and we know through having explored our own body that if our partner did such and such we would go wild with erotic surrender. How do we communicate this?

1) We can tell him in the moment that we love what he is doing and how we would love it if he would also touch us in such and such way. When he does respond, we give him ample verbal acknowledgement.

2) If speaking in the moment feels like it would ruin the moment, we can speak up about it later, approaching the subject with gentleness and love, and asking him if he'd like to hear about what really turns us on.

3) We can direct his body, tongue, hand or fingers with our own body. Body language is a huge communicator.

4) We can volunteer to self-pleasure in front of him so he can watch us and see what makes our juices flow.

Knowing both our own and his erotic fingerprint (what turns us on) will also help. If both individuals are dominant or submissive, both lovers will have to show much more care in order to be fulfilled. Fulfillment comes from our inner self and no one else. If we make our man into a sex god or sex novice, we limit our orgasmic potential with him. Instead, if we approach him with respect, love and an open heart (which leads to a wet yoni) and invite him to play with us in the art of exchange—versus playing the "I need/want something from you game"—we find that we will have a much deeper experience with our partner, as he will experience the same.

Questions: How do you approach sex? What do you do when you feel your desires are not being met? How do you handle a man's ego?

The Art of Succulent Living invites both partners to accept each other's limitations and creates a space of love and gentleness that extends the invitation beyond the ego/*known* into the mystery of the essence/*unknown*. If we always need to be *right*, and we are willing to compromise intimacy, love and respect for the sake of being *right*, we will find ourselves *right but unhappy*. Instead, if we choose to see where our *knowing* creates a boundary, we will also be able to see how such a boundary blocks the opportunity for growth and new experiences. On the other hand, if we desire intimacy, joy, celebration and connection, we can replace the need to be right with the willingness to accept *what is* and the wisdom of *not knowing*. Incredible lovers are not technically perfect—they are lovers who listen and surrender fully to the silent language of the body and spirit.

Questions: How can you let go of what you know for the sake of experiencing something new, spontaneous and beautiful? How can you step out of your comfort zone? How can you form a deeper connection with your partner?

Monogamy and Polygamy

No exploration of the dance of Shiva and Shakti would be complete without investigating the subject of monogamy (loving one) and polygamy (loving more than one). In order to investigate these traditionally taboo subjects, let us set aside our judgments for a moment and accept monogamy and polygamy as being merely personal preferences. Understanding them in this way allows us to experience greater acceptance and to create more authentic relationships.

To remain in our integrity and power concerning the subject of monogamy and polygamy, we align ourselves with our authentic and deepest truth. Authenticity is the ability to match what is inside of us with what we express externally. Living a succulent life requires us to maintain this internal/external congruency in every moment. The only way to be authentic is to know ourselves, to know what works for us. Once our own inner knowing matches our external actions, our level of freedom and love grows. Self-knowledge, self-acceptance, self-love and accepting the authentic expression of our partner, are the necessary ingredients for creating a succulent life. Monogamy and polygamy is a "swept under the carpet" subject, and when left unaddressed, can create tension in a love connection.

Conflict may occur when a monogamous woman engages with a polygamous man (a man who enjoys having additional partners). What often happens is that this woman imposes her values onto the man and wants him to change to become her one and only. But this can only lead to suppression of his true nature, and sooner or later, his polygamous nature will raise its head in protest and possibly lead to adultery. The same tension happens when a monogamous man chooses a polygamous woman as a partner. Eventually her desire to express her true nature (polygamy) could lead her to act in ways that the man would judge as unacceptable. When we understand the nature of our partner as well as our own, we avoid incompatibility issues that may develop over the long term. When the needs of two essentially different people do not form a harmonious connection, one or both is bound to feel unsatisfied.

> Questions: What is your orientation? What is your partner's? Do they match up? How does your new understanding of the dynamics of monogamy and polygamy relate to your life?

Wholeness Leads to Fearless Loving

In the Art of Succulent Living, we see people as being *whole unto themselves.* Embracing others as well as ourselves as whole allows us to direct our attention and energy towards joy and bliss, rather than towards gaining or proving something. When we feel and live the truth of our own innate beauty, passion, intelligence and ecstasy, then we no longer seek fulfillment through the external (through our partners and experiences). Instead, from this place of acceptance of ourselves and of others, we are free to ask real questions and move forward to creating conscious, loving and supportive connections.

I sense that there will be a time when people will exist beyond the finite limitations of fear: fear of being alone, fear of not finding the infamous perfect partner, fear of not being good enough, fear of betrayal, fear of boredom, fear of what is beyond the norm, fear of break-up, and fear of inevitably being alone again. All of these fears can be overcome by cultivating our self-esteem. Through applying acceptance and authenticity to the Shiva and Shakti dynamics in a relationship, we equip ourselves with skills that lead to fulfilling connections and that nurture our wholeness with fearless love.

Exercise: An affirmation for aliveness

I am a courageous, confident, vibrant being who celebrates all that I am and all of life.

Question: What are your fears about connecting with others?

Everyone Does the Best They Can in Every Moment of their Lives

In the dance of Shiva and Shakti, we often see men and women projecting their pain onto others or feeling responsible for the pain of others. This dynamic is natural, yet it is not conducive to authentic, whole, fearless love relationships. An Art of Succulent Living principle that is very useful for helping us shift away from our fear of *getting hurt by others* or *hurting others* is the principle that *we are only responsible for ourselves*. With this principle, we are never responsible for how anyone else feels or for how they may respond to who we are and what choices we make, nor do we see anyone responsible for the responses we choose when reacting to any person or situation. With this understanding—that no person, place or thing has power over us—we can begin to develop a newfound compassion. This compassion is essential if we are to cultivate conscious relationships that recognize the Shiva and Shakti energy within the human aspects of each of us.

This compassion helps us to see that no person has ever intentionally hurt another person. There are no bad people in this world, just good people who have had bad things happen to them. When we realize this truth, we begin our journey into freedom from painful memories. This freedom leads us to manifesting relationships of the highest potential as we no longer choose to replay our old stories in the context of our present day connections. Being compassionate towards people who are unconscious in their harmful actions does not mean we must continuously accept or subject ourselves to these acts. Instead, we can choose to activate our male essence and protect ourselves, then remove ourselves from situations that are not supporting our fullness. Holding on to negative emotions such as hate, rage, anger, fear, etc. may feel like it serves a purpose. But in reality, housing these feelings only hurts us further. Knowing this deepens our ability to make conscious choices, conscious beginnings, and conscious endings.

> *Questions: Do you still feel hurt by someone? Which negative feelings are you still harboring? Even though you might feel that what they did is not ok, how does holding on to these negative emotions help to heal you?*

Healing the Divine Masculine and Divine Feminine

The healing of the Masculine empowers the healing of the Feminine and vice versa. This is because in truth they are one energy. Humans are a beautiful blend of duality (yin/yang) and unity (oneness). As sensual women (Shaktis), we are free to love life fully and free to empower our brothers (Shivas) with our feminine essence so they too may experience loving life fully. In return, our brothers also teach us about the healing qualities of the masculine essence: presence, conscious action and freedom. The blending of Shakti and Shiva, of yin and yang, results in a woman who lives a truly succulent life.

Men represent the essence of freedom and we can learn this from them. Through accepting our own masculine (Shiva) energy, we heal it and allow ourselves the freedom to love passionately, to move past fear into our own personal power and self-esteem. Masculine energy also centers on action and intellect, whereas the Feminine centers on conception and reception of the body. As women, we can choose to blend our powerful body intuition and synergize it with our intellect. We can receive from the world and we can then choose to act from this place of receptivity. Essentially, how we relate to men is how we relate to our own masculine energy. Do we try to control, manipulate or suppress, or do we celebrate the beauty, the power, and the presence?

> *Questions: What is your relationship to your masculine energy? How does it reflect the way in which you relate to the men in your life?*

Being free to choose anew, we are free to be who we really are, and who we really are is a constant dance of yin and yang, of hot and cold, of soft and hard, of Shakti and Shiva. We are free to live past our definitions into the truth of our spontaneous natures. This truth exists for all, including our brothers, and knowing this, we can mend the illusion of separation between the sexes. Everyone wants to love and be loved, to enjoy life, to be free to express oneself honestly, to live beyond the constraints of old beliefs and move into the freedom of spontaneous, harmonious and balanced succulent living. Understanding all of these Art of Succulent Living philosophies sets the foundation for birthing our emergence as sensual women. Now, we are ready to move into the practical applications of the Jade Goddess teachings, to complete and sustain our powerful and succulent transformation.

CHAPTER QUESTIONS

How has your understanding of men and the masculine energy changed?

How do you connect and relate to your own masculine energy?

How does unifying the forces of Shakti/Shiva, yin/yang help you to create a more succulent life?

PART TWO

The Sacred Teachings
of the Jade Goddess

CHAPTER SEVEN

The Jade Goddess Foundation Practices

Techniques to Awaken and
Hone Our Energetic System

The journey begins
with one small step
that's all it takes to create
a new resonance
Along the way
each step so precious
so huge and perfect
Mindfully I walk
stepping lightly upon the Earth
leaving no mark
other than a gentle sigh
as my toes massage
the skin of our Mother
All too soon
the steps shall transform
into the beats
of my wings
as I lift off
into the wild expanse
of the boundless heavens

CHAPTER GUIDE

I N PART ONE, WE EXPLORED the Art of Succulent Living, a philosophy that touches many aspects of our life. We explored what it is like to live as sensual women in a barren world, the relationship between integrity and power, the philosophy of conscious living, the expanded experience of multi-orgasms and omni-orgasms, and our relationship with the Masculine/Shiva. Now we are ready to explore the Jade Goddess foundation practices, the practical application of the philosophy. The roots of these practices come from a Taoist lineage that is thousands of years old, yet their application in the present remains as powerful as ever, as they prepare the body-mind-spirit to exist on a higher frequency of vitality, bliss and peace. They are essential for our emergence as sensual women.

How to Use This Portion of the Book

This portion of the book is designed to be a self-teaching manual to facilitate the learning and practice of powerful techniques that have been proven to aid in the emergence of our sensual selves. It is important to read through this part of the book slowly, one technique at a time, taking the time to absorb and practice each technique before moving on to the next. If we are already experienced with this material, there is a page guide at the beginning of each chapter to facilitate our navigation through the material. All the exercises are described in full, some with images. There is also additional information in italics to indicate what is happening to us when we do each particular exercise.

I encourage everyone to master the foundation practices before taking on more sexual practices. This will ensure our success in the cultivation of our most potent chi, our sexual energy. Do not feel obliged to read each practice chapter from start to finish. Pacing ourselves, we will experience a gradual, yet powerful transformation.

Introduction to the Foundation Practices

The foundation practices embody a combination of meditation and conscious movements that serve as tools for sensual women. Whether we are seeking better health and a balanced lifestyle or a more profound activation and experience of our own sexual energy these practices, while seemingly simple, are in fact very powerful.

A common misunderstanding that people sometimes have about sexual teachings is that explicit sexual acts equate sexual cultivation. An average person with little or no formal sexual education and a desire to understand sexuality will often quickly jump right to the obvious *juicy stuff* (**aroused practice**) and may have little patience or knowledge of the *non-juicy stuff* (**un-aroused practice**). As sensual women, we understand that sexual energy is an innate part of our being. By the simple practice of moving energy in a non-sexual manner, we can experience profound positive shifts in our sexual experiences.

> *Questions: Have you ever thought of ways in which you might be able to cultivate your sexual energy? In what ways do you think a non-sexual practice might enhance your sexual energy?*

Why Practice Something Non-Sexual if Sexual Enhancement is Desired?

From my experiences of teaching the Art of Succulent Living, I have observed that those who do not have a foundation tend to have less success with sexual practices. Of course, this is not the case for everyone. But I have observed that women who are very ecstatic with their sexual energy yet do not have a strong foundation tend to experience a pattern of imbalance that manifests itself in a variety of forms, from physical illness to premature aging to psychological and spiritual issues. Often, we can reduce or eliminate these symptoms by strengthening the body and its energy systems using the following basic foundation practices.

The Three Foundation Practices: Opening and Protecting the Body During Sexual Practice

The foundation consists of three practices:

- ⬥ The Micro-Cosmic Orbit
- ⬥ The Inner Smile
- ⬥ The Six Healing Sounds

Initially, these practices focus on cleansing, purifying and strengthening the body by releasing trapped heat and gases, transforming negative emotions, and literally reprogramming the way our nervous system receives input. The foundation practices also energize and revitalize our body by helping it to digest large amounts of sexual and other energy, circulating this potent energy throughout the rest of our body (not just our genitals) and storing this energy so it doesn't get lost. The Taoist masters view chi as the key to attaining good health and believe that good health enables us to condense and transform more chi to a higher grade of energy.

Question: What images come to mind when you think about using your own energy to heal, balance and enhance your body?

For those of us interested in living succulently, these practices will give us the foundation we need to handle higher volumes of orgasmic energy/chi. Practicing with sexual energy without the foundation practices is like building a house without grounding wires and a solid foundation. It leaves us vulnerable to short circuits and electrical fires, and if we add more floors (higher inner alchemy practices), the whole structure may even collapse. These basic foundation practices rewire our body and clear both potential and existing blockages so that we can enjoy the fruits of our practice.

The Warm-Up Practices

Before doing the three foundation practices (the micro-cosmic orbit, the inner smile, and the six healing sounds), it is good for us to warm up our body and bring our awareness fully into the present moment. When our body is warmed up and our awareness is centered in present time, our ability to perform the practices increase. Repeat each of the following warm-up exercises three or more times, while keeping in mind that the more often we do the exercises, the more results we receive.

SPINAL WARM-UPS

CRANE NECK

We begin (either seated or standing) by sticking our chin out and moving it in an arc downwards, extending the spine. Next, we roll up through the spine, keeping our chin close to our chest. Exhale as we roll down and inhale as we roll up. Remember: the chin leads down and the head is last up. See fig. 7.1 and 7.2.

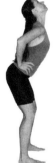

Fig. 7.1
Crane Neck, Exhale

ADDITIONAL CRANE NECK

Twist from the lumbar spine (the lower part of our spine, above the sacrum) to the right and repeat the exercise facing in that direction. Having one hand on our heart and one on our belly is helpful. Repeat this exercise twisting to the left.

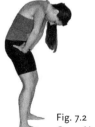

Fig. 7.2
Crane Neck, Inhale

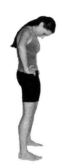

Fig. 7.3
Turtle Neck, Exhale

TURTLE NECK

This exercise is reverse of crane neck. We tuck our chin in and roll down through the vertebrae, sticking our head out of our imaginary shell, then lead with the head as we come up. Exhale down, inhale up. Look at the floor as we roll down, and at the ceiling as we come up. See fig. 7.3 and 7.4.

SPINAL CORD BREATHING

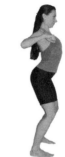

Making our hands into fists and moving our elbows back, we open our chest as we inhale. Let's make sure our tailbone is also tilted back and our chin tucked in. Then we curve forward, tucking the tailbone under and bringing our elbows into our solar plexus, keeping the chin tucked into our chest. On the inhale, open and arch. On the exhale, close and tuck. See fig. 7.5 and 7.6.

Fig. 7.5
Spinal Cord Breathing
Inhale

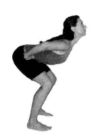

Fig. 7.4
Turtle Neck, Inhale

SPINE SIDEWAYS JIGGLE

Initiate the movement with the coccyx/sacrum (the tailbone and triangular bone connected to it) by wiggling or jiggling it side to side. Slowly continue jiggling from side to side, vertebrae by vertebrae, and making sure they all move. Go all the way to the top of the spine (the base of the skull), then back down. If we have any stubborn areas, we just spend more time there. Inhale and exhale slowly and deeply as we do this.

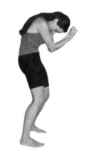

Fig. 7.6
Spinal Cord Breathing
Exhale

HORSEBACK RIDING

This one is done seated on the edge of a chair. Imagining that we are riding a horse and moving our pelvis forward and back, we allow the motion to move up our back. Relax and let the rocking naturally move our spine. Breathe slowly and fully.

All spinal warm-ups will induce a para-sympathetic or relaxation response in our body. These movements encourage the flow of spinal fluid and activate our cranial and sacral pumps. They help to release excess tension along our spine and in our back, enabling us to have better access to the subtle chi movements in our body. Removing blockages in our body will further facilitate the movement of our chi/energy.

Questions: How do you feel after releasing the tension from your spine? How do you see relaxation serving you in your sexual practice?

Beginning the Foundation Practices

Let's now begin the Jade Goddess foundation practices. As with all qi gong energy practice, the results will be equal to the time and energy we invest in them. The first foundation practice is not really a technique so much as it is an attitude. It is the attitude of completely honoring ourselves as sensual women: beautiful, succulent representatives of the Divine Feminine energy. All other techniques stem from this core attitude. To increase the depth of our understanding, the three foundation practices are presented here with theory first, followed by their practical application.

Foundation Practice One: The Micro-Cosmic Orbit Theory

The first foundation practice is called the micro-cosmic orbit. The micro-cosmic orbit is the major path through which energy moves in our body. We all have this orbit; however, it is not fully activated in most of us. Consider our orbit like a super highway and our sexual chi as a fancy sports car. If the highway is covered with roadblocks and debris, we can still get to where we are going, but only if we slow down and take side roads. Before opening our micro-cosmic orbit, however, we will not be able to use our energy (car) to its full potential, and we will not be able to benefit fully from this pathway. When we open and clear this orbit or super highway, we can move our chi a lot more efficiently and effectively. In essence, the micro-cosmic orbit practice is simply placing the tip of our tongue on the roof of our mouth. There are a few different points along the palate where we can place our tongue. I recommend starting with the place that feels the most comfortable.

Exercise: Discovering our palate

By gently curling our tongue back we can feel the roof of our mouth. Finding a comfortable place to rest our tongue allows us to play with this new exercise throughout the day. If our tongue gets tired, we can simply rest, relax and do the exercise again later.

As a result of this practice, we may notice a shift in our energy. In general, the entire body may experience a harmonizing effect.

Shifting Gears

When we become more adept at sensing energy, we can start to move our tongue along our palate until we find a place where we feel some kind of sensation. When we do, we may experience tingling, warmth or electricity, or even taste a metallic flavor. There are typically three main areas of the palate where the tongue is placed. The lung access point is found just behind the teeth and is responsible for moving our energy to the surface of our skin. The heart access point is found on the hard palate and is responsible for moving our energy into our muscles. The kidney access point is found where the hard and soft palate meet. This is the most desirable point to place our tongue, as it moves the energy deeper into the bones and directly connects us to the **crystal palace** (the master glands). When the energy is being transformed properly, a flow of very sweet nectar (saliva) will fill our mouth. See Fig. 7.7.

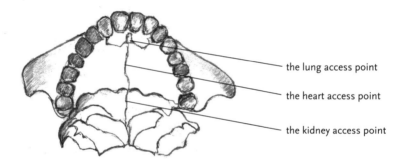

the lung access point

the heart access point

the kidney access point

Fig. 7.7 Sections of the palate to move energy in the body

When this nectar begins to flow, a few things can occur in our body: one, our body's craving for sweets diminishes, and two, our body rejuvenates and regenerates itself.

Mantak Chia emphasizes that, "the saliva is considered a precious fluid in Taoism. It has been called the *Long Life Wine* or *Jade Fluid.*" The more saliva we produce, the better our health will be. Also, Taoists understood that the closer to the teeth we move our tongue, the closer to the surface of our skin our chi will move, the closer to the soft palate (kidney point), the deeper into our body our chi will move. Where we choose to hold our tongue is guided by how we feel and how much saliva we are able to produce.

The other important part of this practice is rooting the feet into Mother Earth. The kidneys and their meridian system are activated through key points:

one, touching our tongue to the kidney point on the palate, and two, being aware of the kidney point on the balls of our feet (called the Kidney-1 or K-1, or the bubbling springs point, see Fig. 7.8). Rooting occurs when our K-1 points are activated by massage, and then through focused awareness of the feet resting on the ground. This is important because the kidneys rule the sexual (Jing) chi in the body, as Mantak Chia confirms, "we believe the kidneys store part of the Original Chi. They also store sexual energy."

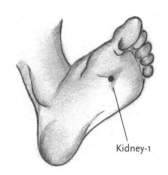

Kidney-1

Fig. 7.8 Kidney-1, bubbling springs point

Another important reason for having our tongue on the kidney point of our palate is that this helps to keep our body cool. This is particularly important because our body generates a lot of heat when doing qi gong practice, more so when we are doing our aroused sexual practice. During qi gong practice having our tongue up on our palate helps us to move the chi from the surface of our body into deeper parts of our body, as we are activating our kidneys which rule the deeper parts of our body.

By using the micro-cosmic orbit to circulate our aroused sexual energy through our body, we not only rejuvenate our body, we also prevent possible imbalances known as the **Kundalini syndrome**. The Universal Tao (Mantak Chia's organization) describes Kundalini syndrome through its symptoms: "Symptoms of Kundalini syndrome: complications that arise because of energy congestion in the head include: sudden baldness, headaches, ringing in the ears, seeing flashing lights, and psychosis."

Important note: We can prevent Kundalini syndrome by practicing the foundation practices described in this book.

> *Questions: Based on what you have just learned about the micro-cosmic orbit, how is this method safer than basic meditation for moving orgasmic energy? How has your view of meditation changed now that you understand its relationship to sexual energy?*

Harmonizing Yin and Yang

The union of the yin (feminine) and yang (masculine) channels (or the front and back channels respectively) is achieved when our tongue is placed on the roof of our mouth (see Fig. 7.9 on the next page). This circuit enables us to move the hot and cold energies throughout the body, removing excess energy from over-heated areas and organs, and redirecting it to areas which are in need of more energy. This in turn creates a greater sense of harmony and balance in our body's organs and tissues. Performing the sexual practices without opening the micro-cosmic orbit can lead to problems as the raw, sexual energy may disperse throughout the body and lodge itself in the organs, tissues or bones creating imbalances. We must always make sure that we refine our sexual energy and give it a direction in which to move. This is very important if we are to fully benefit from our sexual practice.

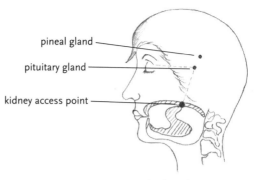

Fig. 7.9 Master glands with tongue on palate

The wonderful advantage to this practice is that it teaches us how to move and direct this energy anywhere in our body, allowing us to benefit from its healing or orgasmic effects. Advanced practices use the orbit for doing energy exchange and for healing others.

Important note: Why do we have to refine our sexual energy? Sexual energy is like raw fuel. When it moves up our spine, it becomes refined into a subtler energy that can be used by our brain.

Foundation Practice One: The Micro-Cosmic Orbit Practice

Now that we understand why the micro-cosmic orbit is an essential part of sexual practice, let's do this practice. We will begin with a pre-meditation warm-up:

Exercise: Warming up before meditation
Let's shake our body and release any tension we might have. It's great to loosen our clothing and do some spinal cord warm-ups (pages 93-94).

ACTIVATION OF EACH POINT
We begin by sitting comfortably on the edge of a chair—planting our sit-bones firmly on the seat, rooting our feet into the Earth (touching the floor)—and by bringing our awareness to our perineum. Our perineum is located between our genitals and our anus, and we activate it when we squeeze the muscles used to stop our flow of urine. We imagine a golden ball of light forming there, and we breathe into this ball of light for a few moments until we feel our perineum grow warm. If we want to create more sensation, we can squeeze and release our perineum.

Then we inhale and bring this ball of light up to our tailbone and leave it there, holding our breath for just a moment. Then we exhale and bring it back down to our perineum. We can do this several times until we feel comfortable with this movement of our attention and energy. We continue by inhaling again to our tailbone, bringing the ball to our sacrum and holding it there, then exhaling, we bring it back down to our perineum.

By continuing with this pattern, we can activate and open each point along our micro-cosmic orbit, using the pattern of inhaling the ball up, holding it for a moment, then returning the ball to our perineum.

Inhale to each of the following points along the yang or back channel:

 ✦ tailbone
 ✦ sacrum
 ✦ door of life or **meng mein** (across from our belly button, in the back)
 ✦ **T-11** (across from our solar plexus in the back)
 ✦ wing point (between our shoulder blades) at T-4 and T-5
 ✦ **C-7** (the big bone that sticks out at the bottom of our neck when we bend our head forward)
 ✦ jade pillow (occipital ridge)
 ✦ crown (**bai hui** point: we can find this point by placing our thumbs in our ears and letting our middle fingers touch on our crown)
 ✦ mid-eyebrow point (ajna)
 ✦ palate

Once we have opened each point along our yang channel, we make sure the tip of our tongue is on the roof of the mouth, and this time, instead of exhaling back down the spine to the perineum, we exhale down the front or yin channel. We do this by bringing the ball of light from our mid-eyebrow to our palate, then down from the tip of our tongue. Then we move it into our throat and each of the points along our yin channel.

Exhale down through each of the following points along the yin or front channel:

 ✦ throat (thyroid and parathyroid glands)
 ✦ thymus gland
 ✦ heart center
 ✦ solar plexus
 ✦ navel
 ✦ sexual palace
 ✦ perineum or **hui yin** (found between the vaginal opening and the anus)

When we reach our navel point, we can continue down to our sexual palace and return the ball back to our perineum, or we can stop at the navel and collect the chi.

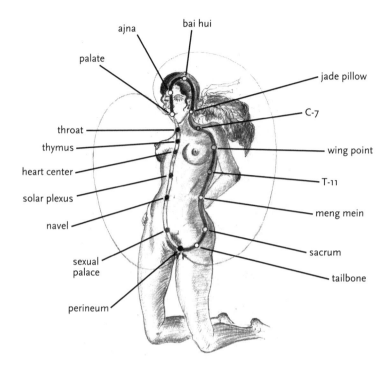

Fig. 7.10
Micro-cosmic orbit points

FULLY ACTIVATED ORBIT

Once we have practiced moving the chi ball from point to point along our orbit, we are ready to move our energy through our fully activated orbit. We begin to do this by inhaling up our spine (no need to stop at any of the points), holding our breath at the top while spiraling the chi/energy like a top in our brain, around the master glands (these glands are referred to as the Crystal Palace in Taoist qi gong). Then we exhale down our front channel. This process of breathing in, holding, then breathing out slowly and smoothly is the practice of moving our energy through our fully open micro-cosmic orbit.

We may experience tingling, warmth or other sensations indicating the movement of energy through our orbit, or we may feel nothing at all. We must not be attached to experiencing these sensations in our meditation as some never happen and some are temporary. However, we will know our orbit is activated when we feel more harmonized, balanced and energized, either in the moment or throughout our day.

Helpful Hints for Successful Practice

✧ We activate each point by touching each one with our finger tips or lightly tapping them.

✧ Activating the yin channel even more as we exhale, our finger tips can trace the channel: starting at the tip of our nose then running our fingers down the midline of our body.

✧ If we cannot feel the orbit or specific points on the meridian, taking the time to meditate just on those points until we sense them will help to open them up.

✧ We must also make sure we are breathing with our belly and not our upper chest.

Safety tip: Having our tongue on the roof of our mouth will act like a grounding wire and ensures that our energy is moving properly. Some of us experience headaches when moving energy through the orbit. This is due to chi staying in our head. If this happens, we can simply focus on our navel and brush our hands down the front of our body. This helps our chi move back down our front line to our navel.

Jade Goddess Orbit Practice

As we do all the practices presented in this book and as we journey deeper into the cultivation of our succulent life, we can remember to keep our tongue lightly touching the roof of our mouth at all times. The more we do this, the more our chi will be able to circulate. This is a very important point to remember, especially when we feel a lot of energy being generated in our body and our yoni.

Questions: Were you able to feel energy moving in the orbit? If you did not feel any energy, have you noticed a change in your overall wellness after practicing this meditation over a period of time and what are those changes?

Storing the Chi

The following step, storing the chi, is the most important step in all the practices and it allows us to fully benefit from the practices.

Breathing into our navel center, we visualize a lasso or spiral of energy moving counterclockwise around our navel. We continue to breathe normally and smile down to our navel as we spiral three, nine or thirty-six times counterclockwise. Then we reverse the spiral, three, nine, or twenty-four times clockwise. Once we are done spiraling, we imagine the collected chi moving into our **cauldron**, which is located at the secondary navel chakra or 1.5 inches below the navel and a few inches inside our body. We form our energy into a pearl and leave it there for future use (see Fig. 7.11).

Spiraling counterclockwise will draw in the chi/energy from all parts of our body, while spiraling clockwise will condense the chi/energy into a smaller and smaller ball of light or a pearl. This is the most important part of our practice.

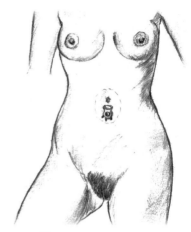

Fig. 7.11
Cauldron for storing chi

Like a rechargeable battery that doesn't keep its charge, even after twelve hours of recharging, our body does not benefit from our practice if we do not make a habit of storing our chi.

Foundation Practice Two: The Inner Smile Theory

The inner smile meditation is the second of the foundation practices and is equally important for the exploration of our sexual potential. As women we typically know more about the outer world than our own body, and often trust experts (such as doctors, therapists and scientists) to tell us what is going on internally after only a five to ten minute examination. How can these professionals really know what is going on inside of us? They can only give a professional and intuitive guess. By relying on these experts, we have come to lack the ability to know ourselves from the inside out. The Jade Goddess teachings help us to get back in touch with our inner wisdom. From this place of knowing our innermost selves, we can collaborate with health professionals in the goal of maintaining our vibrant health.

Questions: How well do you know your body and all its organs and systems?
What is the value in accessing this knowledge?

The inner smile helps us to build a strong relationship with our physical body and increases our ability to understand its language. This simple practice of smiling inwardly to ourselves is actually designed to create a mind-body connection to our internal organs and chi. The inner smile also cultivates our ability to redirect our senses inwardly which increases sensitivity and awareness of the subtle movements of energy within our body. In turn, this helps us to develop an ultra-sensitivity to our body's orgasmic activity.

The ability to direct chi enables us as sensual women to move our orgasm from our genitals to any part of our body that needs healing or activation. That said, *just smiling inwardly* is one of the simplest and most powerful meditations I've come across. The ability to internally transform energy is one of the most important skills for cultivating renewed aliveness in our lives. By making a regular practice of converting external stimulus into internal vitality, we will be well on our way to emerging as vibrant, sensual women.

The inner smile makes us more receptive, more aware, and thus more capable of expanding our experiences. The more relaxed and receptive we are, the greater our pleasure and experience will be.

Foundation Practice Two: The Inner Smile Practice

Our power to deepen our capacity for intimacy through the practice of the inner smile is an essential part of our sexual cultivation. There are a few different stages to this practice that can be done either separately or together.

Exercise: Warming up before meditation
Let's shake our body and release any tension we might have. It's great to loosen our clothing and do some spinal cord warm-ups (pages 93-94).

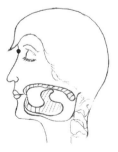

Fig. 7.12
Ajna or mid-eyebrow point
with tongue on palate

ACTIVATING OUR GLANDS
We begin the inner smile meditation by closing our eyes and imagining a person we love, or ourselves, grinning at us. Feeling the warmth of this smiling energy touch our face, we relax our face fully. We draw in more smiling warmth into our **ajna** (mid-eyebrow point, see Fig. 7.12). Allowing our mouth to curve into a soft smile, we feel the smile enter the center of our brain and light up our crystal palace (master glands). Letting the smile

continue down into our mouth, we swoosh it around with our saliva and swallow the mixture, following it with our mind as it goes down into our throat.

We continue smiling into our thyroid and parathyroid glands and we imagine them growing warm, soft and bright. Smiling down to our thymus gland, we watch this gland drink in our smiling light, then open and blossom like a beautiful flower. We can stay here for a moment until we really sense the thymus smiling back at us.

ACTIVATING OUR ORGANS

We continue our inner smile meditation by smiling down from our thymus into our heart. We feel our *heart* soften and relax as the warmth of our

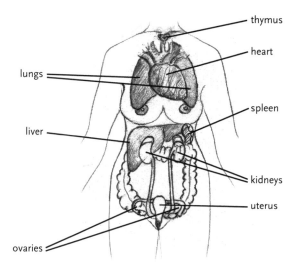

Fig. 7.13
Smiling to the organs

smile beams into it. Sensing if there is any tension, *hastiness* or *apathy* in our heart, we then send the warm, bright light of our smile into those places and observe them transforming into *love* and *joy*.

We then move down to the left, lower rib cage and smile into our *spleen*. Sensing for any *stress* or *anxiety*, we beam the warm, bright smiling light into those places and transform them into *openness* and *centeredness*.

We then continue smiling, moving into our *lungs* and smiling into any areas of *sadness* or *depression*, transforming them into *courage* and *self-confidence*.

By bringing our warm smiling light down into our *kidneys*, we warm them up, transforming any *fear* or *mistrust* into *gentleness* and *calmness*. We can spend some extra time here really making sure the kidneys are warm and smiling.

Finally, we move into our *liver* (located in the lower right rib cage) and sense for any *anger* and *greed*, allowing the warm, smiling light to transform those places into *kindness* and *generosity*.

Returning once again to our *heart*, we feel all the virtues mix in our heart with even more smiling light (love, joy, openness, centeredness, courage, self-confidence, gentleness, calmness, kindness, and generosity). Transforming all the virtues into the super virtue of *compassion*.

Feeling the bright gold-pink light of compassion growing in our heart, we then spiral it down to our *genitals* and wrap every part of them with the bright light of compassion. If we sense any *resentment, frustration, hurt* or *scars* of any kind in our genitals, we can smile into those places. Beaming the healing light of compassion into all those places, we watch them transform into *vibrant, creative energy*. Staying here and smiling softly, we feel our genitals become warm and open.

ACTIVATING THE REST OF OUR BODY
At this point, we may either choose to end the meditation or we may continue on through the entire digestive system (the mouth, throat, stomach, small and large intestines, rectum, and anus) and the entire nervous system (the entire brain, brain stem/spinal cord, and all the nerves throughout the whole body). To do this, we simply smile into each part until we feel them relax and grow warm.

ENDING THE INNER SMILE
Feeling our whole body alive and open, we can bring our smiling light into our micro-cosmic orbit and circulate the smiling energy. It is important to store the chi at the end of our practice.

THE JADE GODDESS SMILE
Simply smile, all the time, during our practice and throughout day.

STORING THE CHI
See page 102.

Foundation Practice Three: The Six Healing Sounds Theory

The third of the foundation practices is the six healing sounds. This practice uses sound vibration and visualization to eliminate stagnant chi (negative emotions) and excess heat from our organs. Just as an overheated car will start to malfunction or breakdown, the same happens to our organs. If our heart is overworked or overheats regularly, after time it will cook itself and be unable to properly perform its function. In addition to treating this problem, the six healing sounds are also a very powerful way for us as sensual women to reclaim the power we have lost through emotional imbalances.

Roadblocks to Enlightenment and Bliss

Any person on the path of higher sexual alchemy and enlightenment may encounter a few roadblocks. For men, it is usually their ego, but for us women, it is usually our emotions. Innately, we feel that it is our right to feel the entire range of our emotions, and we are absolutely correct. However, when the feeling (which is actually a pure message) turns into an emotion (or a distorted message) and we hang on to the emotion instead of acknowledging it as a message, we get stuck. It would be like walking down the road of life and not only stopping to read every single sign along the way, but also pulling it out of the ground and placing it on our back. The load gets heavy fast. The six healing sounds enable us to simultaneously feel the message from our body and release it.

STORY: The power of the six healing sounds

I was driving along to a client's place one afternoon when I suddenly became intensely depressed, so much so that I found myself imagining driving off the road. I knew this was not me, and that my lungs were unbalanced, so I did the lung sound for ten minutes. This cleared the depression and left me feeling cleansed and back to my healthy state of being. No journaling, no girlfriend chats, no counseling. Sometimes our emotions are simply signs of an imbalance. Doing the healing sounds will help us regain balance.

One of the best ways to clear negative emotions is by first doing the six healing sounds (or the one or two healing sounds that relate to the current emotion or emotions we are feeling), then transforming whatever isn't cleared by the sounds by doing the inner smile. Once we are centered, it is easier to examine the situation from a more detached point of view of a witness rather than from an emotionally overwhelmed state of being. This allows us to see where it was that we forgot to love ourselves.

Nevertheless, sometimes we do need to talk to a girlfriend or professional help or a walk or a hot bath. Whichever method we choose to heal ourselves, we can remember to more fully participate in our healing by doing our Jade Goddess foundation practices. We will be surprised at how much faster we are able to come back to feeling centered and free, full of life and enthusiasm.

Often the root of stress is caused by emotions that are felt but suppressed. This type of experience is especially common now at a time when we are more aware of our heads than our bodies. Stress causes our internal organs to over-heat. But prolonged over-heating can lead to the degeneration of the organs and our emotional natures. The six healing sounds release the excess heat and return our organs to a natural state of balance.

Foundation Practice Three: The Six Healing Sounds Practice

The six healing sounds perform the vital function of clearing stagnant chi/ negative emotions from our organs to prepare our body for the amplifying power of sexual energy. The most important part of this practice is the *sound* itself. The vibration (sound) gently releases trapped heat in the corresponding organs. The postures enhance the release of the chi while the visualization of the colors and virtues further deepen the practice.

We begin the six healing sounds by first doing just the sound while visualizing its corresponding organ. Once we are comfortable with that, we may add the posture, colors, and virtues. Below, I present the sounds in the order of the **Creation cycle**. Doing them in this cycle enables our organs to support and enhance each other. However, the sounds can be done in any order.

LUNGS - the Hsssssssssssss sound
Posture: arms above the head, palms turned up, looking up.
Breathe in: visualize a brilliant white light; feel courage and self-confidence.
Breathe out: Hsssssssssssssss, visualize the color gray; releasing depression and sadness.

KIDNEYS - the Choooooooo sound
Posture: hands on knees, back rounded in C-shape looking straight ahead.

Breathe in: visualize the color blue; feel gentleness and calmness.

Breathe out: Chooooo, visualize the color black; releasing fear and cold.

LIVER - the Shhhhhhhhh sound

Posture: clasp hands overhead, palms away, lean left, stretch out the right side, look up.

Breathe in: visualize the color green; feel kindness and generosity.

Breathe out: Shhhhhh, visualize the color brown; release anger and greed.

HEART - the Hahhhhhhhh sound

Posture: clasp hands overhead, palms away, lean right, stretch out the left side, look up

Breathe in: visualize red color; feel love, joy and compassion.

Breathe out: Haaaaaaah, visualize rusty red; release hastiness, impatience, and apathy.

SPLEEN - the Hooooooooo sound

Posture: with both hands, fingers inward, press under the front left rib-cage; lean forward into fingers.

Breathe in: visualize bright gold; feel openness and fairness.

Breathe out: Hohhhhhhh (gutteral), visualize dirty yellow color; release anxiety and worry.

TRIPLE WARMER - the (S)heeeeeeeee sound

Posture: Press straight down with palms from head to hips, point fingers down.

Breathe in: visualize a clear color; feel all virtues and compassion.

Breathe out: Shheeeee, visualize no color; release excess heat.

STORING THE CHI

See page 102.

Questions: Were you able to connect the sound to its corresponding organ? Did you feel you were successful in releasing trapped energy and transforming your negative emotions? How might this exercise benefit your sexual practice?

After practicing the foundation practices, we find ourselves feeling more balanced and filled with vitality. We can either do practices separately or as a set. If we do them as a set, the best combination is to start with our warm-ups, then cleanse ourselves with the six healing sounds and inner smile. To finish, we do our micro-cosmic orbit meditation. Just as little as five minutes per day can change the quality of our lives for the better. Harmonizing and opening our bodies using these powerful techniques gives us a solid foundation for the cultivation of our sexual energy.

CHAPTER QUESTIONS

Which of the foundation practices are you most attracted to?

Have the 6 healing sounds contributed to your well-being and how?

What is the sensation you experience when you practice the inner smile?

CHAPTER EIGHT

The Sexual Foundation Practices

Techniques to Increase and Cultivate
Our Fountain of Youth

*The dance
goes
on and on*

*around and over
and upside down*

I crave such stillness

sometimes the yearning pulls at my yoni

"Yes, lover, please do take me now!"

sometimes it explodes in my soul

"Let me go so I may feel the wind under my wings!"

*Most times I sit
in the middle
of these
two
and just
smile*

CHAPTER GUIDE

The Jade Goddess foundation practices help us to remain harmonized and balanced in our body-mind-spirit. As we prepare ourselves for the core practices using the Jade Egg, we first must turn our attention to the sexual foundation practices. These techniques are specific for working with our un-aroused sexual energy and are sometimes referred to as the **Fountain of Youth** practices as they help us connect with, increase, and circulate our ovarian energy.

How to Use This Portion of the Book

As with the Jade Goddess foundation practices, the sexual foundation practices section is to be read slowly and thoroughly. Mantak Chia reminds us that the Jade Egg practice was seen "as a great secret taught by the Taoist sages to empresses and concubines, these methods enabled women in an emperor's court to maintain their sexual activity, beauty, and health for a long time." The exercises are given first, with an explanation in italics of what happens when we do the exercise. Let's begin to tap into our innate ability to rejuvenate ourselves through accessing our ovarian energy.

SEXUAL ENERGY PRACTICE WARM-UP

These warm-ups are traditionally done after the regular warm-ups (pages 93-94), and before the Jade Egg practices (pages 140-180). Sexual energy practice warm-ups are a practice in themselves and can be done individually or sequentially.

GENITAL BREATHING

This technique uses five points to bring more chi into our body and to pump up (or activate) our sexual energy. The first two points are at the bottom of our feet, the K-1 (Kidney-1) point, the next two are the center of our palms P-8 or **Lao gung** (see fig. 8.1), and the fifth point is our perineum.

Imagine that we can drink in chi from these points (alternatively, we can also project chi outwardly from these points). As we inhale, we feel like we are drinking or sucking in the Earth chi through all five points. As we exhale,

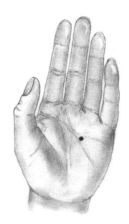

Fig. 8.1
P-8 or Lao gung point

we send that chi into our pelvis, warming our genitals. Simultaneously we thrust our pelvis forward slightly on the inhale and backwards on the exhale. Our breathing rate should be medium to quick. Repeat this nine to thirty-six times. Then we continue with the following technique.

This exercise will warm the body and generate a lot of sexual energy. It is great to do before a practice or if we feel low in energy and need a burst of fresh chi.

GROUNDING/EARTH CONNECTION

After we do a series of nine genital breaths, we create a ball of chi at our perineum and hold our tenth breath. Focusing our awareness on our perineum, we feel it grow warm and bright. Then we exhale and split the ball into two, sending it spiraling down our legs into the Earth (screwing/spiraling ourselves into the Earth to feel more grounded). This can be repeated several times until we feel present and centered. We may also want to visualize drinking in the bright blue light of the Earth chi as we relax after the exhale.

This exercise is very grounding and allows us to be more connected to the Earth chi. The Earth energy is very nurturing and sensual and is also empowering for our kidneys and, thus, our sexual chi.

Questions: How do you feel after energizing your pelvis? How can grounding the energy benefit your sexual practice?

KIDNEY BREATHING

Breathing into our feet (through our K-1 point) we connect to the Earth's chi, by first squeezing our perineum on the inhale, then holding our breath as we rub our hands together to create heat. When we exhale, we place our right hand onto our right kidney. Using the fingers of our left hand, we massage our liver (tucked under the lower right portion of our ribcage). With chi fingers (imaginary energy fingers), we imagine reaching and massaging our right kidney while continuing to inhale and exhale, releasing any stuck chi into the Earth. Resting our left hand over our liver, we feel the chi/heat grow warm between our hands. Then we focus on expanding our kidney into the right hand as we inhale and penetrate our kidney with chi on our exhale. We do this for awhile until we feel our kidneys are warm and relaxed. Dropping our hands at our sides, we pause to sense the difference between the two sides of our body, and then we repeat the entire exercise on the other side, this time focusing on the spleen and the left kidney.

This is a very important practice to do when we menstruate, as it will help us to replenish the chi lost through bleeding. This is also great to do if our adrenals are taxed (over-active) and when we are cold or tired.

KIDNEY PACKING

This technique is a continuation of the kidney breathing exercise. In this exercise, we move from kidney breathing directly into kidney packing by changing our breath pattern and staying aware of the Earth's healing blue energy. Packing means holding the breath to energize. This action tells our body that we want it to pay attention and to amplify what we are doing. We begin "packing" by inhaling three times, taking tiny sips of air and squeezing our perineum with each breath. Squeezing once on the right side of the perineum (connected to the right kidney), once on the left of the perineum (connected to the left kidney), and once in the center of the perineum (visualizing both kidneys). We then hold our breath or pack the chi into our kidneys, then gently exhale and penetrate our kidneys with the Earth's healing blue chi.

This exercise further helps the kidneys to regenerate themselves, keeping them strong and vibrant.

NOTE: If we are not used to deep breathing, we may feel dizzy or nauseous as our lungs and body are cleansed and cleared of old, stagnant chi. If we really feel unwell, it is wise to stop for awhile and just practice at a slower pace.

Questions: Were you able to feel warmth in your kidneys? How does kidney breathing affect your overall energy?

PRE-OVARIAN BREATHING

Ovarian breathing begins by bringing our hands down from our kidneys to our ovaries. To locate our ovaries, we place our thumbs on our navel, relaxing our hands (see fig. 8.2). Where our pinky fingers land is where our ovaries are and where our index fingers land is where our sexual palace is found. We place our lao gung point in our palms over our ovaries and we connect our heart to our sexual organs. We then imagine the chi from our kidneys spiraling and wrapping around our ovaries (see fig. 8.3, next page). This is done by

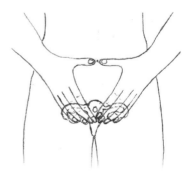

Fig. 8.2
Locating ovaries and sexual palace

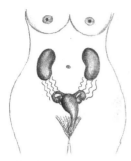

Fig. 8.3
Breathing from kidneys
to ovaries

inhaling to our kidneys and exhaling down to our ovaries. Feel them grow warm and tingly (if we need to, we can rub our ovaries in both directions to stimulate them). Once we can feel this energy relationship between our kidneys and ovaries, we move onto simply inhaling and exhaling to our ovaries.

Special note for women who have had full or partial hysterectomies: All the practices are excellent for reestablishing a healthy flow of energy into this part of our body as well as rejuvenating our glands (for lubrication, etc). Even though the physical structure(s) may no longer be there, we still have our etheric sexual organs.

OVARIAN BREATHING

Continuing from the pre-ovarian breathing into ovarian breathing, we now bring our focus to our **ovarian palace**, which is an energy collection point located in the center of our womb (see fig. 8.4). Connecting with our ovarian chi, we direct it with our intention to move into our ovarian palace. We do this by using our breath. Inhaling, we focus on collecting the ovarian energy from the ovaries,

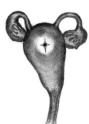

Fig. 8.4
Ovarian palace

and exhaling, we focus on sending the chi into the ovarian palace (see fig. 8.5). To aid in this process, we use our lower belly, extending it out on our inhale and pulling it inwards (creating suction) on our exhale. We breathe and direct the chi this way until we feel our womb get warm or tingly and by keeping our awareness in our ovarian palace until we sense it filling with our ovarian chi.

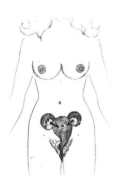

Fig. 8.5
Breathing from
the ovaries to the
sexual palace

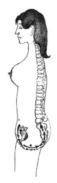

Fig. 8.6
Redirecting the chi
from the sexual palace
into the orbit

Once our palace is full we redirect our sexual energy into the micro-cosmic orbit by sending the ovarian chi down to our clitoris, perineum and tailbone/anus while taking three sips of breath (one to each point). At the tailbone, we hold our breath for a brief moment, then we exhale and send the chi up our spine to our crown (see fig. 8.6). Inhaling, we spiral the ovarian chi in our brain (around the master glands), then we exhale and bring the chi down our front channel. We can choose to either store it in our navel or continue back down to our ovarian palace and allow the chi to move on its own through our micro-cosmic orbit a few more times. We then repeat the whole exercise.

This exercise helps to activate our ovaries and ovarian chi. Breathing in this way gives a sensual woman greater access to the powerful ovarian chi and its rejuvenating properties. It also provides us with a way to rejuvenate our glands and enliven ourselves. Doing ovarian breathing along with breast massage (as described in Chapter 11) may affect our moon-time (menstrual period) by reducing PMS, cramping, and other uncomfortable symptoms of chi stagnation in our genitals.

NOTE: Do not do this if you are pregnant or wearing an **IUD**.

Questions: Were you able to feel the ovarian energy? After an extended period of practice, what benefits of mastering ovarian chi have you noticed for yourself?

OVARIAN COMPRESSION

This exercise can be done directly following the ovarian breathing. We begin by inhaling into our throat centers and imagining a golden ball of chi forming there (see fig. 8.7). We then hold our breath and swallow this chi ball down, feeling it move down past our solar plexus and navel (see fig. 8.8) and into our ovaries. Continuing to hold our breath in our ovaries and feel the chi ball in our belly pushing down towards our ovaries while we pull up on our perineum (see fig.8.9). This compresses our ovaries and packs them with chi. Normally, we hold our breath for twenty seconds or less.

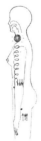

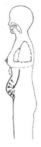

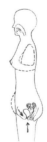

Fig. 8.7
Swallow the chi ball

Fig. 8.8
Chi ball moving
down to belly

Fig. 8.9
Chi ball moving
down to ovaries

As we feel the need to breathe, we take a second sip of breath and compress our ovaries again by gently feeling the chi ball pushing down while we pull up on our perineum. Then we exhale up our spine, sending the chi into our micro-cosmic orbit once again. Once our chi is in our brain, we inhale and spiral the chi around our master glands, then exhale down to our navel. We must run our orbit (feel the energy move through our micro-cosmic orbit) a few times in between compressions.

Doing genital breathing between each round allows us to catch our breath.

NOTE: If we feel dizzy or unbalanced, we can twist our waist to the right and left a few times and then brush the energy down from our head to our navel.

ALTERNATIVE ADDITION FOR OVARIAN COMPRESSION

We can also do this exercise with our legs positioned in a **horse stance** (with our feet placed wider than hip width apart) and with our upper body bent forward with our back flat like a tabletop (see fig. 8.10). We begin by inhaling in this tabletop position and holding our breath while doing the compression exercise. When we need to exhale, we then stand straight up and let the chi rise up our spine to our brain. This may cause our ovarian chi to rise quickly. Do not continue if there is any discomfort. Also remember that the downward pressure on our ovaries is done with our chi, not with our muscles.

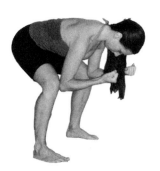

Fig. 8.10
Horse stance with table-top flat back

*This intense exercise enhances our ovaries and our ability to access our ovarian chi. As noted by Mantak Chia, "this exercise reduces mental problems, strengthens the ovaries and the cervix, and increases the power of the vaginal muscles." We may feel dizzy or buzzed as the chi rushes up to our brain. If we feel really light-headed, focusing on our navel or K-1 points on the soles of our feet or placing our hands on the floor will help. This exercise also activates our **throat chakra**, connecting both our throat and our **sex chakra** in a powerful way. This connection of our creative expression center and creative power center is profoundly healing for our sexual energy. They are yin and yang to each other and whatever condition one center is in, often the other center will be in a similar place (for example, if we feel that we have throat issues such as speaking our truth, quite often there is a similar* *energy blockage in our sexual center. Opening and healing one of them starts the healing process for the other).*

NOTE: Do not do this if you are pregnant or wearing an IUD.

Questions: Were you able to connect with the chi released from the ovaries in this exercise? How do you view your relationship between your throat and sex center?

UPWARD DRAW (YIN/YANG)

This exercise uses our micro-cosmic orbit path in our body to pull our sexual chi away from our genitals and move it up to the brain. As the chi moves from each point along the micro-cosmic orbit channel, it opens the orbit even further while refining our raw sexual chi into a more subtle sexual chi that our brain can then absorb and use to rejuvenate our entire body. There are two kinds of upward draws: the yin (gentle) way and the yang (strong) way.

YIN: Doing nine or more genital breaths (see genital breathing, pages 115-116), we then create a ball of chi at our perineum and hold the energy there for a moment. We sip (inhale) the ball of chi up our spine (we can choose how many sips and points along the back channel of the micro-cosmic orbit to sip to). Holding our breath, we spiral chi in both directions around our master glands/brain, and then we exhale down our front channel to our navel. We can brush down the energy to our navel if necessary.

YANG: Doing nine or more genital breaths (see genital breathing, pages 115-116), we then create a ball of chi at our perineum and hold the energy there for a moment. Next, we exhale up our spine making the lung sound (hsssss) at each station (or at least a few key ones) until our lungs are empty. Holding our empty breath, we spiral the chi around in our brain. Continue spiraling in the brain and inhale, then release the breath and chi down the front channel to our navel. We can brush down the energy to our navel if necessary.

NOTE: You can choose to repeat both or either with the tabletop, flat-back position.

This exercise prepares us for moving fully aroused sexual energy through our micro-cosmic orbit. We may find that moving warm or semi-aroused chi in this way will be really invigorating and rejuvenating. If we practice this while engaged in intercourse or aroused sexual practice, we would use the upward draw before orgasm occurs as a way to continually circulate our aroused sexual chi from our genitals into the rest of our body. This will enhance our sexual experience as well as potentially lead us to experiencing a full body orgasm.

NOTE: If we practice the upward draw with a non-practicing partner, there is a possibility that we may draw up their chi as well, depleting our partner. It is best to do this exercise when we are not connected at the genitals or when our partner is also practicing the sexual techniques.

Questions: Were you able to draw the aroused energy away from your yoni into the orbit? How did this feel when you did this?

Complementary Practices

After doing the sexual energy warm-ups, the complementary practices can be added to enhance both our awareness of our sexual chi and its cultivation.

NEUTRAL PRACTICE

This is the practice of stopping and doing a non-judgmental scan of where we are at on all levels of our body, mind, emotions and spirit. This enables us to track if and when an emotional or physical reaction to the practice might occur. Developing a way to witness our reactions during practice is essential as many of us instinctively stop when we feel pain (emotional or physical) or go into the energy of the imbalance instead of using those experiences to inform us of when we may need to do our own self-healing.

Self-healing is a major component of the Jade Goddess teachings. It plays a vital role in increasing our capacity to be fully independent, alive and succulent. As sensual women cultivating our practice, we become aware that, contrary to popular belief, a man or partner is not solely responsible for our orgasm, but that we ourselves are fully orgasmic beings able to share our orgasmic energy at will.

SEXUAL REFLEXOLOGY

Reflexology works by connecting the massaged point on the reflex zone to our nervous system. In his research study, Dr. Piquemal was able to demonstrate a statistical correlation between five selective reflexology areas of the feet and the dermatomes of the nervous system (dermatomes are innervation of skin segments based on fetal development). Another study by Terry Oleson, PhD, and William S. Flocco was done using an analysis of reflexology as a means to reduce PMS symptoms in women. They found "a significantly greater decrease in premenstrual symptoms for the women given true reflexology treatment than for the women in the placebo group."

Sexual reflexology works in a similar way to traditional foot, hand and ear reflexology, except that it is a unique practice involving the reflex zones of our genitals.

The main difference found between traditional reflexology and sexual reflexology is that sexual reflexology affects not only the organs of our body, but also our energy systems. For example, the kidney zone in the vagina affects the entire kidney system including the physical organ, the meridians of the kidneys, the bladder meridians, and the bladder itself. Another difference lies in its practical application. Traditional reflexology uses massage of the feet, hands and ears, whereas sexual reflexology relies on isolating contractions of the vagina and occasionally internal massage of our reflex zones.

In the practices of the Jade Goddess teachings, we use an innovative combination of traditional Taoists practices to further enhance the potency and effectiveness of this practice. Here we blend the wisdom of sexual reflexology with the cleansing power of the six healing sounds. This unique combination is profoundly powerful, and very effective in releasing blockages, energetic or physical, in our yoni. This exercise may be practiced either with or without the Jade Egg (see Jade Egg practices in Chapter 9). It is also a fantastic practice to do before and/or after sex.

REFLEX ZONES

The following section introduces each of the reflex zones of our vagina and their relationship to both our body and our emotions. The way we practice sexual reflexology is by connecting with each zone and sensing what is going on for us in both that area and in the rest of our genitals. Then we inhale and imagine the positive color and virtues bathing the tissues of our genitals while squeezing the zone of our choice. Exhaling, we release the negative color and emotions. We do this three or more times, then we rest and imagine again the positive color and virtues filling our genitals. We can slowly move from zone to zone, or just do the area that needs the most attention.

KIDNEY ZONE
Located at the opening and the first segment of the vagina.

The negative aspect of kidney is *fear* and *doubt*. We may experience fear when our yoni's are exposed or touched. Exhale the negative emotions and the color *black* with the chooo sound.

The positive aspect of the kidney is *gentleness* and *calmness*, qualities that are characteristic of a sexually open and confident woman. Inhale *blue* with the positive virtues.

LIVER ZONE
Located at the middle and 2nd segment (the G-spot area) of the vagina.

The negative aspect of liver is *anger* and *greed*. We may experience anger when our yoni's **G-spot** is massaged or touched. Exhale the negative emotions and the color *brown* with the *shhhh* sound.

The positive aspect of the liver is *kindness* and *generosity*, qualities that are characteristic of a woman who feels full and abundant sexually. Inhale *green* with the positive virtues.

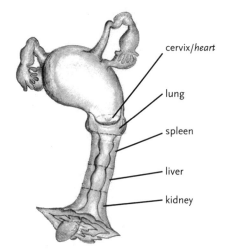

Fig. 8.11
Sexual reflex zones

SPLEEN ZONE

Located at the top and 3rd segment of the vagina.

The negative aspect of spleen is *worry* and *anxiety*. Deep penetration can sometimes cause us some anxiety or to worry about how we look, etc. Exhale the negative emotions and the color *dirty yellow* with the *hoooooo* sound.

The positive aspect of spleen is *openness* and *fairness*, qualities of a woman who is centered in her sexual power. Inhale *gold* with the positive virtues.

LUNG ZONE

Located at the top or shelf area of the yoni and the area around the cervix.

The negative aspect of lung is *sadness* and *nostalgia*. This is often the most neglected area of a woman's genitals and, when stimulated, this zone can activate feelings of sadness or nostalgia. Exhale the negative emotions and the color *grey* with the *hssssssss* sound.

The positive aspect of lung is courage and self-confidence, qualities connected to a woman who lives fully in the present, free of her past. Inhale brilliant white with the positive virtues.

HEART ZONE

Located at the cervix itself.

The negative aspect of heart is *hastiness* and *impatience*. We may experience this in sexual encounters that are not of an open-hearted nature.

Exhale the negative emotions and the color rusty red with the *haahhhhh* sound.

The positive aspect of heart is *love* and *joy*, attributes of a healthy connection between our sexual center and our heart. Inhale *ruby red* with the positive virtues.

Extra on the heart: When our cervix is overly banged on, it may lead to our hearts energetically shutting down and provoking a "hurry up and get off me" feeling.

This entire practice of using sexual reflexology with the healing sounds is an integral part of the cultivation of our sexual energy. Whenever we have intense emotions that come up, especially in sexual experiences (alone or with another), sexual reflexology with the sounds is a powerful tool for transforming our negative experiences into vitality.

SACRED YONI MEDITATIONS

PINK PEARL MEDITATION

This meditation is done either at the end of the sexual foundation practices or at the end of our Jade Egg practice.

We begin lying down or sitting and focusing our chi in our perineum. Here we create a beautiful pink pearl and visualize it spinning there, feeling it pulsate brightly. Gently we bring the pink pearl to our inner labia and imagine sipping or drawing it up into our yoni. We then feel the pearl slowly spiraling up our vaginal canal, painting our vagina with soft pink light, moving slowly upward. Once at the top (the cervix), we reverse the spiral and move back down our vagina. We repeat this until we feel our entire vagina is bright with pink light.

We are now ready to move the pearl to the mouth of our cervix. Imagine our cervix is sipping in the pearl. We then spiral the pearl in our womb and paint the walls of our womb with bright, soft pink light, covering our entire womb. Continuing, we split the pearl into two pearls and move them into our fallopian tubes and paint those with soft pink light. Bringing the pink pearl to our ovaries, we also paint them with bright, soft pink light. We end this practice by bringing the two pearls back into one pearl and sending it back down through our vagina and into any part of our body that needs love and healing chi. We rest feeling our genitals bright, healthy and vibrant, making sure to collect and store the chi once we are finished.

This meditation is used to heal and activate our genitals. It promotes a refined connection with our sexual selves.

FIGURE EIGHT MEDITATION

This meditation is also done either at the end of the sexual foundation practices, at the end of our Jade Egg practice, or after the pink pearl meditation.

Beginning lying down or sitting, we focus our chi in our perineum and feel our pearl (our chi) forming. We then bring the pearl to our inner labia and

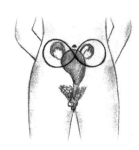

we gently sip it up into our vagina, slowly spiraling it around, moving it up and down a few times, and massaging all sides (visualize painting the tissue with a pink light). Now, we imagine that we are playing a very gentle game of ping-pong with the pearl, lightly tapping and activating all of the bliss-spots throughout our yoni.

After tapping our entire yoni, we sip the pearl up into our **uterus** through our cervix, repeating both the spiraling and the gentle ping-pong inside our womb, activating and painting her in pink light.

Fig. 8.12
Figure eight around the ovaries

Now we begin the figure eights by spiraling the pearl to each ovary and creating a figure eight around them, with the sexual palace in our womb being the center of the eight (see fig. 8.12). Once we are comfortable with that figure eight, we can continue creating figure eights around the throat, navel, breasts and heart, and any other combination we feel drawn to do.

We collect and store the chi when we are finished.

This meditation is very powerful. Remembering to keep our tongue up, we make our breath full and slow. If there is a lot of energy in our genitals, we can sip it up the spine, spiral it around in our brain, then bring it down to our navel. Moving our chi through our orbit allows our entire being to be washed with this fountain of youth elixir.

Questions: Were you able to sense this imaginary pearl? Were you able to feel the figure eights? Which one felt the most healing to you?

STORING THE CHI

This exercise is identical to the Jade Goddess foundation practice found on page 102.

REST-YIN PRACTICE

All the techniques shared thus far are part of the do-ing or yang part of our practice.

Yin practice is done to create balance by focusing on be-ing. This is done immediately after any practice by spending anywhere from a few minutes up to a half hour resting and doing nothing, simply feeling the results of our invested effort.

This yin element of the practice has equal importance for our wellbeing as this is when the body begins to assimilate the changes and to integrate all that was experienced. It is in doing nothing that everything happens.

The experience of cultivating our sexual energy through the sexual foundation practices is sufficient for beginning our transformation process as sensual women. The practices prepare our bodies for the potent practice of the Jade Egg, while giving us more vitality, balance and a sense of self-mastery.

CHAPTER QUESTIONS

What value—physical, emotional, mental, spiritual—do the sexual foundation practices have for you?

Which one of the sexual foundation practices appeals to you most? Which one was the most difficult to understand or experience?

After several months of practicing the sexual foundation practices, what changes have you noticed in yourself? In your sexual energy?

CHAPTER NINE

The Core Jade Egg Practices

The Secret Teachings
of the Jade Egg

Warrior Princess
there is no Prince Charming to kiss
and wake you from this deep slumber

only you hold the power to choose

so wake now Goddess
seize your passion-flame by the core and hold on
for this moment is now of pure stillness

a pause
the Universe holds its breath
awaiting your choice
awaiting like the tall columns on either side of
the gateway, pillars to the portal of life

wake now sweet goddess
for your sleep has been full and long

Life is calling
seeking to activate your inner truth
spread your wings, oh great fire dragon
Free yourself from the illusions of fear
a rich and vibrant path is inviting you

Now is your moment

Will you take that giant step off
the cliff and leap into the wisdom
of the
Great Unknown?

CHAPTER GUIDE

Now that we have built a strong and clear foundation, we are prepared in our body-mind-spirit for the core of the Jade Goddess teachings: the Jade Egg practice. The Jade Egg itself is a key instrument in the art and mastery of cultivating our sexual energy and its practice comes from a lost lineage of powerful women, the lineage of female Taoists. The wealth of the Jade Egg practices that follow come from my distillation of key pieces of wisdom that have been passed down to me by various teachers and from the careful attention I've paid to my own inner guidance and wisdom. Through sharing these secret teachings with women around the globe, I have been able to further test and confirm their effectiveness and truth. I only teach that which I do myself; therefore, all that follows is tried and true.

How to Use This Portion of the Book

As with the two foundation practice chapters, the Jade Egg practices are meant to be experienced like a gourmet meal: slowly enough to appreciate all their subtleties. It is important that we take our time with each exercise, relaxing into connecting with our bodies in this new way. Getting to know ourselves intimately is a life-long journey.

It is important, at this point, to encourage the practice of both the sexual foundation techniques and the care of our yoni and breasts (as explained in Chapter 11) as they are essential to our success with the Jade Egg. To familiarize ourselves with our sexual anatomy and the use of sacred sexual language (yoni, sacred temple, etc), I have included thorough information on these topics in Chapter 11. The more holistic an approach we take towards harnessing our most potent life force, the more success we will have. Remembering also to trust and relax into the unfolding of our lives serves us greatly as we venture into this ancient form of energy cultivation.

To make the best use of this chapter, we must take our time to thoroughly read the exercises and their explanations (in italics) a few times before attempting to do the practice. We should also stop immediately and rest if we feel any discomfort or pain when attempting to do the Jade Egg practices. However, before jumping into the practices, a little practical information on the Jade Egg itself will facilitate our preparation.

The Jade Egg Theory

What is the Jade Egg?

One of the greatest tools we can use to enhance our sensual life is a Jade Egg. It is a piece of natural jade (nephrite or Jadeite) that is carved into the shape of an egg and then drilled from top to bottom. The following quote addresses specifically why a green Jade Egg is our preferred egg of choice when first starting our Jade Egg practices. Acupuncturist Andrew Pacholyk states,

> "Jade is considered the health, wealth and longevity stone, and is used for increasing our courage, wisdom, emotional balance, stamina, love, humility, generosity, peace, and harmony. Jade is also known as being androgynous: therefore, it is considered to have a gentle, steady pulse of healing energy and helps us rid ourselves of negative thoughts and energy. It is also very beneficial to our heart in both a physical and spiritual sense and is a very protective stone, keeping us as the wearer out of harm's way. Green Jade is the most common of all Jade and is particularly calming for our nervous system, helping us channel our passions in a constructive way, making our expressions of love easier."

In China, where this practice has its roots, a wonderful myth exists that describes Jade as being the solidified semen of Dragons. According to this myth, jade is seen as a pure form of yang chi and when we place it in the most yin part of our body it is thought to create a harmonious balance of the yin and yang energy within us.

Jade is an ideal tool as it is one of the harder crystals and will not break as easily if boiled or dropped. After we sensual women have used Jade for many years, we may then choose to upgrade to an obsidian egg, then to a rose quartz egg. Some of us may not follow this belief and may choose to use any egg we please. I trust each woman knows best for herself and I can share a personal experience to demonstrate the intensity of the rainbow obsidian egg.

STORY: *Uncovering the potent power of the black egg*

A senior instructor and colleague in the Universal Tao system had a supply of obsidian eggs and gifted me with one along with this warning: "This egg is many times more powerful than the Jade Egg for cleaning the yoni. Be aware of this when you use it." I proceeded to use the egg and within a couple of hours I started to experience a bizarre discharge. When tested, this discharge was nothing a modern doctor could recognize. I felt the power of this egg and chose to go back to my Jade Egg until my body healed more thoroughly.

The same instructor shared, "Once the obsidian egg has purified the yoni, then a woman can graduate to the rose quartz. This has the frequency of love. It is important to be really clear before using the rose quartz, so as not to grow negative energy patterns." I thanked him and smiled, acknowledging the mystery of this practice.

My experience with the obsidian egg was very powerful. Since it is volcanic rock (hot yang fire coming from the depths of earth), it is best used only when we have sufficiently attained a high level of harmony and balance in our body-mind-spirit. This level of practice is beyond the scope of this book.

The Benefits of Using a Jade Egg

When considering this practice some of us may experience some apprehension or fear. This is a natural response to something we do not understand. In the Jade Goddess teachings, using the Jade Egg is an invitation, not mandatory. Trusting our innate wisdom and inner guidance will allow us to begin this practice on our own time. The benefits of these exercises are numerous, ranging from the purely physical to the spiritual or energetic. Many of my students have benefited greatly from doing the practices without the Jade Egg and once they felt ready, the Jade Egg has helped them reach the next level of their exploration and cultivation of their sexual practice.

Question: How do you feel about the idea of using a Jade Egg internally?

The Joy of Dexterity

On the physical side, the Jade Egg is an excellent tool for exercising our vagina and pelvic muscles. By vaginally moving the Jade Egg, we develop our strength and suppleness, and we are able to notice an increase in our sensitivity to sensation and pleasure. This is due to our increased dexterity. This also has positive effects for our partner. Our yoni's increased dexterity allows us to literally suck or pull our partner's finger, tongue, or penis into ourselves, literally enabling us to play them like a flute.

One of the great benefits of dexterity for a heterosexual couple is that when our partner has a soft penis, our increased dexterity will allow us to fully pleasure ourselves (and, in effect, our partner) by moving his soft penis around using the muscles of our yoni. This takes the pressure to perform off our partner and allows him to relax into the new possibility of soft penetration. For some of us sensual women, a softened penis can be much more pleasurable than a fully engorged one as we can do much more with it and thus stimulate ourselves more.

Another benefit of dexterity is that it enhances solo and same-sex cultivation.

A dexterous and powerful yoni enables us to access a greater range of orgasmic responses even when we have nothing inside of us. Just a few squeezes in the right places and we can become aroused very quickly. Whatever our sexual preference, having awareness and control over our own pleasure and orgasmic potential creates more and more joyful and ecstatic experiences for all involved.

Question: Does the concept of developing vaginal dexterity for increasing sexual and sensual pleasure fit with your idea of sexuality?

STORY: *Increasing our natural lubrication*

One woman who attended a short introduction to the Jade Goddess teachings said that she always had to use a lot of lubrication because she had difficulties becoming wet. After the class, she bought an egg and went back to her cabin to play with it. The next morning she came up to me and shared that she had never been so wet in her entire life! She was so excited and grateful.

Using the egg helps to increase vaginal secretions and to activate the bartholin's glands (the glands that lubricate the vagina).

The Energetic Side of Practice

Along with its powerful physical effects, the Jade Egg also has an effect on the energy of our yoni. Using the egg enables us to access our sexual reflexology zones, bringing more energy/chi to the various organ systems in our body (for more on sexual reflexology, see Chapter 8). As sensual women, we can add the use of our Jade Egg to our sexual reflexology practice to activate a whole body experience of our sexual energy, with or without orgasm. This practice also further enhances clearing negative emotions stored in our sexual tissues.

The Jade Egg practice keeps our sexual energy circulating throughout our body instead of allowing it to become stagnant or congested in our genitals. Frigidity, over-arousal, and other sexual issues can often be traced to either the repression (stagnation) of sexual energy or over-stimulation (depletion). Using the Jade Egg enables us to access our creative/vital life force consciously and helps us to direct this life force to any part of our body for healing or activation.

STORY: *Mastering our sexual energy*

Personally, using the Jade Egg has enabled me to redirect my sexual energy in such a way that I have been able to not only reap the benefits of better health, but to also create the life I want. Prior to the Jade Egg practice, I felt scattered and unclear, although very passionate and full of energy. I like to use the analogy of a horse-drawn carriage. If twelve horses are all pulling the carriage in different directions, we will not get too far. Sexual practice is about getting all our horses to point in the same direction, while Jade Egg practice gives us the ability to control the reigns.

Another benefit to the Jade Egg practice is our ability to access greater amounts of sexual chi and to use it for transformation on physical, emotional, mental, and spiritual levels. When we are able to contain this energy in our body (like a sealed jar), without any leaks and cultivate it (so the jar is always full), then we can choose when, where, and with whom the contents will be shared.

> Question: Knowing that the Jade Egg practice is used to activate and move your sexual energy to affect your entire body, how would this shift your current ideas and habits of sexual expression?

Enlightenment Fuel

For a moment, let's consider our sexual energy as being the rocket fuel to our enlightenment. If this is indeed the case, then learning to access and direct this energy can play a powerful role in awakening our consciousness. If the idea of spirituality and sex does not fit into our perception of reality, we may simply prefer to use the Jade Egg practice as a key for accessing our potential as a sensual woman. If we aimlessly squander and pour out our fuel (sexual energy), we will not have enough for lift off when the time comes, nor will we be able to attain our hidden dreams and goals as easily, if at all.

> Question: Has spirituality ever been a part of your sex life?

Redefining Orgasm

As we examine the multiple applications of the Jade Egg, from gross physical exertion to subtle chi movement, we begin to see a new definition of orgasm emerging. According to its traditional definition, the orgasm is limited to a physical description: muscular contractions in the genitals and pelvis accompanied by a flush of hormones. By using the Jade Egg, we can access many more layers of orgasm.

Those of us who say we have never had an orgasm have most likely had one, though perhaps not in the traditional sense of the word. We are actually capable of experiencing much more subtle expressions of bliss such as the sensation of tiny bubbles rising through our body. If we consider the subtlest expression of orgasm as the release of energy during our DNA's replication process, then, each cell in our body must experience this orgasmic delight of creation as it duplicates itself. With up to a hundred trillion cells, that is a lot of mini-orgasms! These sensations, however, are so subtle that unless we have our awareness developed enough to sense these tiny movements of chi or bliss-gasms, they may go on unnoticed.

The lack of subtle awareness is a result of an over-stimulated culture. Everything has to be *big*. *Big* breasts, *big* vajra's (penis), *big* bank accounts, *big* adventures, *big* dramas. Seldom do we investigate and experience the subtleties of our life. Cultivating our energy through the Jade Goddess foundation practices enables us to be more and more aware of subtle movements of chi, whereas using the sexual practices enables us to trace and activate the ecstatic energy that our body continually generates.

> Questions: *When you experience orgasm, do you feel that it is not just physical, but also subtle in its manifestation? How does the awareness of having mini bliss-gasms throughout your entire body help you to understand yourself as an orgasmic being?*

Our Clitoral System

One wonderful benefit of using a Jade Egg is that it helps us access the greater sexual potential that lies dormant in our pelvis in what is called our **clitoral system**. Our **clitoris glans** (the sensitive tip we can easily see and touch) is only a small (but important) part of the extensive and interconnected network of tissues, blood vessels and nerves that we call our clitoral system. In her book, *The Clitoral Truth*, author Rebecca Chalker, gives a detailed description of all the muscles surrounding the vaginal canal and how they are interlinked with the clitoris. As the tissues and muscles of our yoni get stretched and squeezed, they send signals through our clitoral pleasure system that enhance our arousal sensations. The more we use the Jade Egg, the more chi and blood we bring to our clitoral system. This, in turn awakens our limitless pleasure system.

The Perks of Regular Practice

Just as those of us who brush our teeth regularly have less dental issues than those of us who do so sporadically, those of us who consistently practice with the Jade Egg reap the benefits of healthy sexual organs and open, expressive sexual energy. However, when starting any new exercise program, it is important to do only as much as is reasonable. The same goes for the cultivation of sexual chi. Sporadic practice is better than no practice at all. This is where our personal wisdom and internal guidance will help us to set the pace and regularity of our sexual practice.

The Ancient Wisdom of Sexual Power

Why are the teachings of the Jade Goddess secret? The ancient Taoists knew that anyone who had awareness and control of their vital essence could be very powerful and could even create *anything* they desired. This is why in ancient times these practices where only given to royalty (so they could rule longer) and to the lineage of Taoists that would continue to preserve the tradition. These secrets were not intended to be common knowledge and students were chosen wisely and carefully so as to avoid the possible misuse of power. The Jade Goddess teachings were born of the secret teachings of the ancient Taoists. Now, however, they are openly shared with any woman who chooses to practice the Art of Succulent Living. To prevent misuse of the teachings much attention is given to the activation and development of our heart, the seat of compassion.

Process versus Goal-oriented Practice

The Art of Succulent Living and the secret teachings of the Jade Goddess are considered to be a process-oriented path. This means that on this path our focus is on where we are right now rather than on where we should be. When exploring the following practices, a light-hearted, fun attitude will lead us to success. Rather then attaining any specific goal, this practice is geared towards the gentle unfolding of our inner wisdom and innate succulence as women.

Process-oriented practice indulges in the moment, in the sensations currently being experienced, instead of focusing on a desired sensation (which is goal-oriented). Like walking up a mountain towards the peak, the goal-oriented focus plows forward, keeping our attention firmly locked on the idea that the peak is our goal. On the other hand, the process-oriented focus takes in all the sights along the way, loving them and enjoying them and perhaps deriving so much joy from them that reaching the peak is of little importance. Sex is not meant to simply be about attaining our biggest and best orgasm, which is a goal. It is about exploring our creative life force while playing in the realm of ecstatic adventure, which is an unfolding process.

The Secret Jade Egg Techniques

Now that the reasons for practicing with the Jade Egg are clear, let's move into doing the practices by setting up a time with no disturbances and creating a safe space to explore these sacred teachings. If we do not yet have a Jade Egg, we can still do the exercises by simply using our imagination or, for those of us who are comfortable with touching ourselves, using our finger in place of the Jade Egg. In fact, I recommend all sensual women to occasionally use our fingers instead of our egg as a way to feel what is happening to our muscles and to receive direct **bio-feedback** on the progress of our practice.

Preparing Our Jade Egg

Prior to beginning the Jade Egg exercises, we need to prepare our egg by boiling it for ten minutes to sterilize it. Note that this only needs to be done before the first use and occasionally as maintenance or if we drop our egg. After our Jade Egg has cooled, we thread some non-waxed, non-flavored dental floss through the hole in the center of our egg. The Jade Egg is drilled for easy threading and easy removal, and for the practices that require a counter force and for the more advanced techniques of using weights (as in **bone marrow nei gong**). Some women opt to use light-weight fishing line or organic cotton string which is easy to clean between uses.

When we are ready to use our Jade Egg, we place it in our underwear, pants, or skirt to warm it against our belly. When using the egg, we always make sure the knot is on the outside of the body so as to prevent irritation.

Important Tip: Before we begin these practices, it is best to do the warm-up exercises (see Chapter 7 and Chapter 8).

Our navel center, also known as the lower **tan tien** (or elixir field), is the safest place to store all the energy we generate during practice. Any time we feel overwhelmed, simply focusing on our navel or the soles of our feet and brushing down from our head to our navel with our hands will help us feel more centered and relaxed.

JADE EGG PRACTICES: LYING DOWN

PRE-INSERTION PRACTICES
CONNECTING OUR HEART TO OUR WOMB
Beginning on our back, we place our left hand on our heart and our right hand on our womb/belly and rest for a moment. We release three *Haahhh* sounds, bringing the love and warmth of our heart down to our womb. We begin by inhaling to our heart, feeling love and warmth, then exhale down to our womb, feeling it warm up. Next, we create a cocoon of light around ourselves, feeling it surround us with a sense of safety and warmth. We then ask permission of our body to do the Jade Egg practice. If we get a no, we honor that and do our practice at another time. If we get a yes, we are ready to move on, always remembering to listen to our own inner wisdom and guidance. No matter what practices we perform, we recognize that we

do know what is best for us and we honor that. Sealing our commitment to listening to our inner guidance, we do three more *Haahhh* sounds and then rest for a moment.

WARMING MASSAGE

With our Jade Egg still warming against our belly (or in a cup of warm water), we rub our hands, exhaling the warmth and love of our heart into our hands and then we start to massage our belly. Feeling for any areas of tension, pain, sensitivity, or coldness, we smile into those areas as we gently and firmly massage ourselves in a manner that feels good for each of us. We keep breathing deeply and slowly into our belly as we massage around our ovaries and womb, imagining long chi fingers going deep inside of our belly, we release any tension that may be blocking our flow of chi.

While continuing our massage, we gently squeeze our mound of Venus (pubic bone), our qua (groin area), and our inner thighs (see fig. 9.1), sending love and appreciation to them, recognizing their strength and power. This activates our spleen, liver and kidney meridians, helping us to increase our sexual energy. Next, we roll to one side and massage around our anus (also known as our love muscle). We then send warmth and love to this important muscle. Continuing on to our perineum (also known as the gate of life and death) we release any tension we find there. Finally, we massage around the bony structure of our yoni and our **outer labia** itself. Toxins may be stored in our fatty tissues and this massage helps to release

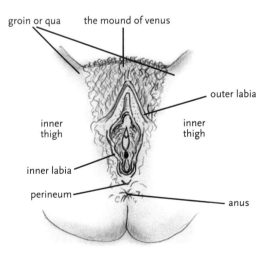

Fig. 9.1
Female genitals

the stored toxins in our blood and flush them out through our elimination system. Our intention during this exercise is to release any blockages in our body through massage and to prepare our body for moving our sexual energy. This important step also helps to create a healthy communion between ourselves and our genitals.

The more blood that flows into the area, the more chi, arousal and sensitivity we will experience.

CONNECTING OUR HEART TO OUR YONI

Placing our left hand on our heart and our right hand on our yoni (see fig. 9.2), we rest for a moment and then release three Haahhh sounds, bringing our love and warmth from our heart down to our yoni, feeling our yoni warm up. If we sense we need to do a few more Haahhh sounds, then we take the time to do this now.

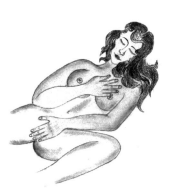

Fig. 9.2
Heart-yoni connection

More practice tips:

✧ Remembering to keep the tip of our tongue on our palate during all of the following sequences of exercise will enable our energy to move through our micro-cosmic orbit as we practice.

✧ Remembering to smile throughout our entire practice will keep our heart soft and open and keep our body receptive and aware. This also seals our gate of life and death (perineum or hui yin).

✧ All of the following exercises can be done without a Jade Egg, however, the practices are more effective with it.

SUCTION POWER

INSERTING THE EGG

You may choose to use a personal lubricant if you do not find yourself sufficiently self-lubricated after doing the sexual foundation practices.

Once we feel ready to begin inserting our Jade Egg, we take our egg and place the larger end on the inside of our inner labia. We may choose to keep one hand on our heart to remind ourselves of the heart and yoni connection. Gently we move our egg in a circle and slowly search for the best angle for our egg, where it feels like it just fits (see fig. 9.3 on page 143).

When we have found the right spot, we rest there and do another three Haahhhh sounds, bringing more love and warmth to our yoni.

This very sweet practice allows us to honor the sacredness of our yoni and to truly listen to when we are ready to receive the egg/finger/lingam.

Question: *How does the egg feel to you? Notice all your feelings and sensations throughout these practices as they will guide you perfectly.*

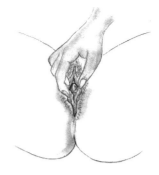

Fig. 9.3
Resting with the egg in the inner labia

SIPPING

As we inhale, we gently sip or squeeze the tip of our Jade Egg with our inner labia. Upon exhaling, we relax our grip and feel our vaginal canal yawn open. What we are doing is creating a vacuum that will suck in our egg. We do this until we feel our egg start to move inwards. We can apply a very light pressure with the hand that is holding the egg to encourage it to move inwards, taking our time, and never forcing our egg in. Our yoni loves to be entered gently, with love and honor. We keep breathing deeply and stay connected to our heart. Once we feel complete with this exercise, finish off with the following cum-passion exercise.

Sipping will start to activate the kidney system that will further activate the sexual energy/ovarian chi. It also develops the idea that sex can be gentle, nurturing and profound. Anatomically, it exercises our **bulbocavernosus muscle** *(see fig. 9.12 on page 152).*

CUM-PASSION

This exercise is a key component of the Jade Egg practice. It is done at the end of each exercise. To begin the cum-passion exercise, we rub our hands together and exhale the warmth and love of our heart into our hands. Massaging our ovaries in circles, moving in both directions, we imagine that we are collecting our ovarian chi and bringing it up into our breasts by pulling our hands up the mid-line of our body to our breasts (see fig. 9.4). Then we massage our breasts in both directions. This stimulates our heart to transform the sexual chi into more and more compassion.

This powerful practice transforms raw sexual energy into the

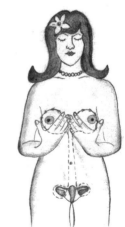

Fig. 9.4
Cum-passion chi

more refined and magnetic healing energy of compassion. As we develop sexually, we simultaneously nurture the development of our heart chi (love, joy and compassion).

Since this is so important, I have placed a short reminder after each of the Jade Egg exercises to encourage us to do this practice regularly. It will appear as such:

CUM-PASSION (Repeat to cultivate more compassion chi).

REST

Occasionally, it is important we rest and simply be aware. This is an important part of the practice as it enables us to cultivate the yin aspects of who we are. Let us practice resting and simply being aware now.

As this practice is also essential for our cultivation, I have place a short reminder after each of the Jade Egg exercises to encourage us to do this practice. It will appear as such:

REST (Repeat for yin chi cultivation).

SIPPING WITH PELVIC ROCK

Doing the same "inhale-sip, exhale-yawn" movement that we did in the sipping exercise, here we add a very gentle pelvic rock. Inhaling, we rock our tailbone upwards towards the ceiling, making sure we do not lift our pelvis off the floor (we just aim our tailbone *up*). Exhaling, we rock our tailbone down towards the floor (our back will arch a little bit). Inhale-sip-*up*, exhale-yawn-*down*. Moving gently and sensually, we enjoy the movement. The slower we breathe, the more exquisite it becomes.

This rocking motion activates our sacrum and cranium pumps and moves our sexual energy/chi up into our orbit. It also releases any back tension (which may be blocking our chi from moving) and allows for naturally pleasurable movements to manifest within our body.

CUM-PASSION (Repeat to cultivate more compassion chi).

REST (Repeat for yin chi cultivation).

SIPPING WITH PELVIC TILT

This exercise is the same as the sipping-rocking exercise, only this time we keep our pelvis tilted up towards the ceiling (with our back flat on the floor) for *both* our in and out breath. Inhale-sip-*up*, exhale-yawn-*up*. This will help to pull our Jade Egg in deeper. The more we can relax on our exhale, the more our egg will be pulled in. Once the egg is inside, we rest for a moment.

This exercise opens our mid-back further and helps us to access our T-11 pump (located across from our solar plexus, on our back). It also strengthens our muscles by incorporating dynamic tension with slow breathing techniques.

CUM-PASSION (Repeat to cultivate more compassion chi).

REST (Repeat for yin chi cultivation).

PELVIC POWER

STRENGTH AND SUPPLENESS

Placing our feet flat on the floor and bending our knees, we inhale, lifting our pelvis up off the floor as far as we can while squeezing our yoni/egg tightly (see fig. 9.5). Exhaling, we roll down through our spine slowly, relaxing the squeeze and releasing the *mmmm, ooooh* or *aahhhh* sounds (see fig. 9.6). Inhale-up-*squeeze*, exhale-down-*relax* and moan. We do as many as we like (normally three of each sound is good). We rest by pulling our knees to our chest and relaxing our back.

Moaning opens our throat chakra, enabling our sex chakra to further open and activate. The sex and throat centers have a yin and yang relationship. This means that if one is blocked, the other will be blocked too. Moaning also helps us to spread our chi throughout our body instead of just keeping it in our genitals.

CUM-PASSION (Repeat to cultivate more compassion chi).

REST (Repeat for yin chi cultivation).

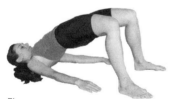

Fig. 9.5
Press up and squeeze while inhaling

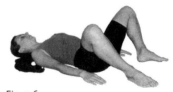

Fig. 9.6
Relax down and moan while exhaling

GROIN STRETCH

While lying on our back, we bend our knees toward our belly and grab our ankles or shins (which ever is more comfortable) and gently stretch out our groin/qua. If we like, we may add a slight rocking motion side to side. *This exercise helps to increase the suppleness of our inner thighs and hips, further enabling the sexual energy to be moved throughout our whole body. It also allows our whole body to connect our pelvis.*

CUM-PASSION (Repeat to cultivate more compassion chi).

REST (Repeat for yin chi cultivation).

EGG PUSHING

With our feet flat on the ground, we gently rock our pelvis, but again this time, as we inhale, squeeze hard on our egg while tilting our tailbone up. As we exhale, we push down as if we are having a bowel movement and tilt the tailbone down. Our egg should move up and down in our vaginal canal. Inhale-squeeze-*up*, exhale-push-*down*. We do not push so hard that our egg comes out.

This exercise strengthens the muscles we use during an A-frame orgasm. An A-frame orgasm is also known as a G-spot orgasm and results in the upper muscles of our vagina tightening and pushing down while the opening of our vagina relaxes open. This exercise also helps our body to understand the unique mechanics of female ejaculation and trains us to bear down and out instead of pulling in and up during orgasm.

CUM-PASSION (Repeat to cultivate more compassion chi).

REST (Repeat for yin chi cultivation).

ROCK AROUND THE PELVIC CLOCK

Lying with our feet flat and knees bent, we locate our sacrum (the triangular bone at the base of our spine) and imagine that 12 o'clock is the top of our sacrum. This would make 3 o'clock the right side (back hip), 6 o'clock the tailbone, and 9 o'clock the left side (back hip). Starting at 12 o'clock, we press this top part of our sacrum onto the floor while keeping our back flat. We then roll slowly towards 3 o'clock, then down to 6 o'clock (tailbone). Our back should now be arching. We then continue rolling to 9 o'clock, and then back to 12 o'clock. Moving slowly in a continuous circle, we go both clock-

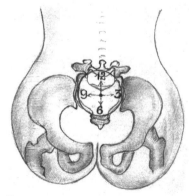

Fig. 9.7
Rock around the pelvic clock

wise and counterclockwise. If we find any parts of our body feeling blocked or stiff, we just go more slowly through those parts. By breathing with our belly slowly and by smiling into the sacrum, we make our movements luscious.

While this is not an egg-focused exercise, it is important for activating our sacrum. It will also further allow our body to release tension held in the sacrum, pelvis, and lower back area. If we indulge in the sensuality of this exercise and bring our awareness inwards, this exercise can also teach us how our subtle pelvic movements can activate different muscles and sensations, thus increasing our ability to access bliss.

Special Note: As stated by Mantak Chia, "The coccyx and sacrum are the gathering centers of all major nerves and are closely connected to the organs and glands. (When they) are open and connected, one feels balanced; when closed, one feels imprisoned." *Doing the Rock Around the Pelvic Clock exercise helps us to open our sacrum and coccyx, thus promoting a more balanced, harmonious experience of our sexual energy.*

CUM-PASSION (Repeat to cultivate more compassion chi).

REST (Repeat for yin chi cultivation).

ROCKING INTO THE EARTH

Lying with our feet flat and knees bent, we place our hands with our palms down onto the floor. Starting with the in-breath, we inhale while digging our fingers and toes into the floor and feel our back arch, pressing our tailbone into the floor (see fig. 9.8). Then, we exhale while pressing the soles of our feet, the palms of our hands, and our back into the floor, tilting our tailbone up (see fig. 9.9). Next, we gently inhale and repeat the exercise, pulling the chi into our body during our inhale and pressing the chi deep into our body during our exhale. We can then reverse our breathing pattern and keep our body movement the same: inhale and press, exhale and claw. During both methods, we make our movement as sensual as possible.

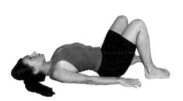

Fig. 9.8
Rocking into the earth while inhaling

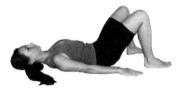

Fig. 9.9
Rocking into the earth while exhaling

Indulging in this is a highly sensual experience that has the potential to induce much pleasure as it involves our whole body moving and blending our sexual chi of our yoni with the sensual chi of the earth. Enjoy!

CUM-PASSION (Repeat to cultivate more compassion chi).

REST (Repeat for yin chi cultivation).

SPINAL RELEASE WITH PULSING

Lengthening our legs until our heels are pressed into the floor, we begin by keeping our knees slightly bent. We start to pulse our feet (move them forward and back, pointing and flexing) and allow that motion to move our spine along the floor, forward and back. Totally letting go, we relax, feeling the spinal fluid activate. This will feel effortless.

This exercise further activates the movement of our spinal fluid leading to deeper relaxation. This is key to experiencing orgasm and bliss and also releases any blocks or tension held along our entire spine.

CUM-PASSION (Repeat to cultivate more compassion chi).

REST (Repeat for yin chi cultivation).

BUTTONS OF BLISS (REMOTE CONTROL)

Buttons of Bliss is a series of exercises designed to develop our connection to our perineum area, linking it with our internal organs and select meridians of our body. It is also called the remote control because once mastered, we can move our chi anywhere in our body through the activation of the different buttons or points around our perineum, thus remotely affecting the selected area of our body with our sexual chi.

LEFT AND RIGHT ACTIVATION

Straightening our legs completely and bringing them close together so that our ankles are touching, we begin by pointing one foot while flexing the other, slowly alternating right and left. Bringing our awareness to our vaginal canal, we imagine that the movement of our feet actually initiates from the left and right sides of our vagina. Placing our fingers just above our pubic bone, we point them inwards towards our vaginal canal, creating a mind-body connection.

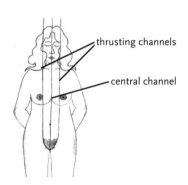

Fig. 9.10
Thrusting channels

This exercise activates the right and left sides of our yoni, thus activating the right and left thrusting channels in our body. These thrusting channels are part of our body's energetic system and they run parallel to each other (see fig. 9.10). They originate from either side of our perineum and terminate in our skull, on either side of the Bai Hui point (crown point). They are responsible for bringing energy to our different vital organs as well as to our brain.

Activating these channels gives us greater capacity for self-healing and for the cultivation of bliss as a whole body experience. As we get used to moving the right and left sides of our yoni, we are able to direct our energy/intention to either side of our body. This is how we start to redirect our orgasm into the rest of our body. This exercise is very effective at toning the muscles of our vagina.

CUM-PASSION (Repeat to cultivate more compassion chi).

REST (Repeat for yin chi cultivation).

WINDSHIELD WIPER

In this exercise, we move our legs so that when we turn our flexed feet in towards each other our big toes touch. Then we rotate our feet away from each other, keeping them flexed. It is easier if we keep our legs straight for the entire exercise so that we can become aware of the front and back of our vaginal canal. We then rotate in and relax, then rotate out and squeeze our gluts and yoni muscles. We repeat this inward and outward movement of our flexed feet as much as we like, keeping our movements slow and remaining aware of the movement initiating from inside our vagina.

These movements exercise the front and back parts of our yoni. This helps to further activate the micro-cosmic orbit channels and has a firming affect on our yoni.

CUM-PASSION (Repeat to cultivate more compassion chi).

REST (Repeat for yin chi cultivation).

5 BUTTON REMOTE

This practice specifically activates the five points that are connected to our perineum (see fig. 9.11). These five points are the remote control of our body as they enable us to start moving our energy and awareness to different regions of our body. This is very energizing and healing for each region related to the activated point.

The first point is our clitoris. It is responsible for activating our pineal gland and opening the front channel of our micro-cosmic orbit. The sec-

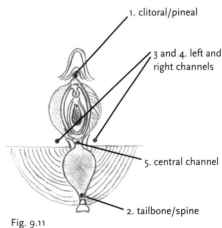

1. clitoral/pineal

3 and 4. left and right channels

5. central channel

2. tailbone/spine

Fig. 9.11
5 buttons of bliss

ond point is our tailbone and the back part of our anus. It is responsible for opening up the back channel of our micro-cosmic orbit. The third and forth points are found on the left and right side of our perineum. They activate the thrusting channels of our body. The final point is our perineum itself. It is responsible for activating the central channel that runs straight up from the middle of our perineum to our crown point in the skull (Bai Hui point).

1. CLITORAL/PINEAL CONNECTION

Locating where our outer labia and pubic bone meet, we feel around with our finger until we locate our clitoral ligament, which feels like a tight rubber-band. Pressing firmly down on our ligament, we start to pulse or squeeze it (up and down, rather than side-to-side). Later, we will be able to isolate the ligament independently, but at first we will feel like everything in our pelvic area is squeezing all at once. If this happens, we just relax and remember to breathe from our belly. As we practice, we get used to isolating the clitoral ligament from the rest of our genitals.

During this exercise, we become aware of the connection between our pineal gland and our clitoris. This opens the front channel in our body, activating our master glands and our crown chakra: in effect, spiritualizing our sexual practice. Orgasm occurs in our brain first. Thus, activating this connection is a great way to induce orgasm and/or deep pleasure.

>   **CUM-PASSION** (Repeat to cultivate more compassion chi).

>   **REST** (Repeat for yin chi cultivation).

2. TAILBONE/SPINE

Locating our tailbone and the back of our anus, we lightly contract and release our anus. We then imagine that we are gently sipping up into our spine. This movement feels like a very gentle pulsing of our anus/tailbone.

Some of us experience significant chi arousal during this exercise, so let's remember to keep our tongue on the roof of our mouth to activate our back channel. Also keeping in mind that we are training our love muscle (anus) to pull our aroused energy up our spine, the more we practice, the more natural and easy this activity feels.

>   **CUM-PASSION** (Repeat to cultivate more compassion chi).

>   **REST** (Repeat for yin chi cultivation).

3 AND 4. LEFT AND RIGHT CHANNELS

Rather than activating our deep vaginal walls (as we have in the previous exercises), this exercise is geared towards finding our transverse muscle. Our transverse muscle lies beneath our perineum and is connected to our sitting bones (see fig. 9.12 on page 152). It activates our left and right thrusting channels.

We begin the exercise by bending our knees and placing our feet flat on the floor. Pressing our left heel into the floor, we then **palpate** the left side of our perineum. The easiest way to do this is to first find our sitting bone and from there move our fingers inwardly towards our perineum. We will need to press firmly inwards as we are doing this because the transverse muscle is located deep inside our pelvic floor and is hard to feel. The movement should feel like we are squeezing and releasing (pulsing) the left side of our perineum. We then repeat this entire process on the right side.

We must remain aware of the left side of our body or our left channel (thrusting route) during this exercise and remember that our thrusting channel starts on either side of our perineum and moves up the inner left side of our body, up to the left of our crown point. When doing our right side, we must then shift our awareness to the right channel (thrusting route). This may cause a different sensation than the deep, internal, vaginal stimulation of the point/flex exercise; however, both exercises access the side channels.

CUM-PASSION (Repeat to cultivate more compassion chi).

REST (Repeat for yin chi cultivation).

5. CENTRAL CHANNEL

For this exercise, we focus our awareness on our perineum as we squeeze, imagining our chi going straight up to our crown point. Then, as we relax, we feel our chi move back down to our perineum. Inhale-up, exhale-down.

This exercise opens and clears our central channel (see fig. 9.10 on page 148). Sometimes our awakened sexual energy (Kundalini) can shoot straight up the central channel which is why we must focus on keeping our tongue up and moving our chi through the micro-cosmic orbit. If we feel dizzy or have a headache afterwards, we must focus on the movement of our chi down the front of our orbit. We also can brush down from our head to our navel, encouraging the excess chi to move back down to our navel center.

Once we have activated all five of our buttons and are able to control them individually, we will find that we are able to move our orgasmic chi

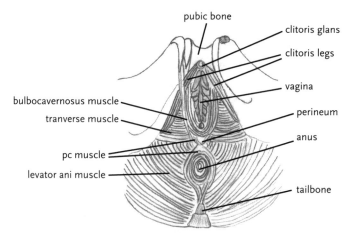

Fig. 9.12
Muscles of sexual anatomy

into any part of our body simply by slightly squeezing any of the places in our yoni or around our anus.

For a more advanced practice, we can feel the chi move in a spiral-like pattern through each of our channels and through our body parts.

CUM-PASSION (Repeat to cultivate more compassion chi).

REST (Repeat for yin chi cultivation).

TURNING OVER, LYING ON OUR BELLY

ROCK AROUND THE PELVIC CLOCK ON OUR BELLY

This exercise is the same as Rock Around the Pelvic Clock (see page 146), except now, instead of lying on our back, we lie on our belly. In this position, we imagine the hands of the clock being at the following new positions: 12 o'clock will be our solar plexus, 3 o'clock will be our left hip, 6 o'clock will be our pubic bone, and 9 o'clock will be our right hip. We now move our hips in a circle in both directions, keeping our tongue up on the roof of our mouth, and our hands placed under our forehead. Keeping our awareness inside our yoni as we circle, we breathe slowly and fully, noticing what is happening internally.

For extra practice, we can also add an exercise called *Humping the Floor*. For this exercise, we press our pubic bone into the floor and then we move our tailbone upwards. Inhaling, we press our pubic bone into the floor, and on the exhale, we press the tailbone back up.

This exercise helps us to massage out any blocks in our belly and spirals our energy up along our spine, further enhancing the movement of our sacrum. If we would like a deeper massage, we can place our fists (or small balls) under our belly, moving them around to different spots.

REST (Repeat for yin chi cultivation).

ALTERNATE NOSTRIL BREATHING

To begin, we turn our head to the right while remaining face down on our belly. The right nostril will be free and away from the floor and the left nostril will be closest to the floor. Closing the left nostril with our left hand, we inhale through our right nostril while we simultaneously squeeze the right side of our yoni and our right transverse muscle. We hold our breath for a moment, then relax and exhale. We repeat this nine times. Then we turn our head to the left side and repeat the entire exercise using our other nostril and the other side of our yoni. We also repeat this nine times. Finally, we place our forehead on our hands and this time we inhale through both nostrils while squeezing our entire yoni. We hold our breath for a moment, then exhale and relax. We repeat the exercise nine times.

This exercise opens our thrusting routes from our feet up to our head as well as our central channel (see fig. 9.10 on page 148). It also helps to balance the energy in our body, while refining our muscular control of the left and right sides of our yoni. Having full awareness of the movement of our energy while resting deepens our experience.

REST (Repeat for yin chi cultivation).

COBRA STRENGTH AND SUPPLENESS

KUNDALINI PRAYER

Lying face down with our palms placed at our shoulders, we curl our toes under so that they rest on the floor. On our inhale we press up gently as far as we feel comfortable and squeeze our Jade Egg tightly (see fig. 9.13). Then we exhale and roll down, one vertebrae at a time, relaxing our hold on our egg and feeling ourselves surrender or melt into the floor. We do this exercise three or more times.

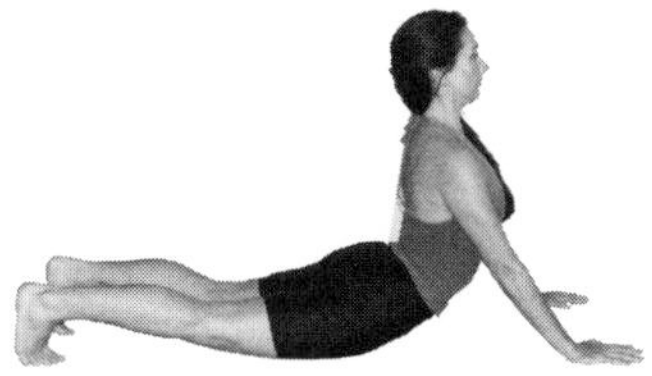

This exercise opens our spine and encourages our sexual chi to rise up our spine to our brain. As we remember to keep our tongue resting on our palate, we also roll our eyes up as though we are looking into

Fig. 9.13
Kundalini prayer while inhaling

our own brain at our master glands on our inhale. We fully relax on our exhale. Inhaling clears our spine and activates our Kundalini or aroused sexual chi. Exhaling moves our chi through our spine and down the front. This may cause us to feel a tingling sensation throughout our entire body.

NOTE: Our micro-cosmic orbit will naturally spill excess energy over into the other channels of our body or into the organs that most need it. We do not have to direct this chi. We can just relax as much as possible and let the intelligence of our body and chi take over.

KUNDALINI PRAYER FOR TWO

This exercise can also be done with our partner inside of us (behind and on top of us). To perform a dual version of this exercise, we both inhale and push up, holding our breath and squeezing together. Then we gently roll down together and exhale. We rest between each lift, keeping our tongues up and feeling our chi circulating.

This exercise is a very sweet and intense dual-cultivation practice. It is ideal for partners that both know how to circulate chi through the orbit. We must make sure that our partner supports their own weight during this exercise.

REST (Repeat for yin chi cultivation).

KUNDALINI PRAYER WITH THROAT ACTIVATION

Inhaling the same way as in the previous solo exercise, we press up and squeeze while tucking in our chin and rolling our eyes up. Now we breathe quickly with our belly, in and out like a pump. This is known as **energizer breathing**. We do this breathing nine times. When we are finished, we inhale a full breath and hold it while squeezing our egg even more tightly. Then we exhale slowly and melt down to the floor while releasing *mmmm*, or *ooohhh*, or *aahhhh* sounds. We do one of the sounds three times, then move on to the next sound.

This intense exercise may induce an orgasm as it moves our sexual chi from our genitals to our pineal/pituitary (master) glands while activating both our throat and sex charkas. Remembering to place our tongue on the roof of our mouth as we inhale will help move the chi. When we relax we keep our tongue up and witness our energy move through our orbit. If we are able, we add a pulsing squeeze of our egg as we hold our breath. This is a very powerful exercise and a long rest period is advised.

REST (Repeat for yin chi cultivation).

LICKING THE MIGHTY ICE CREAM CONE

Starting in a child pose (see fig. 9.14) with our hands stretched out in front of us, we inhale and move towards our hands, keeping our chin close to the floor as long as possible (our butt will stick out during this exercise). We then roll through our spine and press up into the cobra position as we

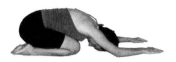
Fig. 9.14
Child's pose

stick our tongue out as far as possible. As we do this, we imagine that we are licking an ice cream cone or a vajra (penis) or anything else we desire imagining. When we reach the highest point of the posture or the end of our breath, we place our tongue on the roof of our mouth and hold our breath for a brief moment while squeezing our egg. Then we exhale and push ourselves all the way back into child pose while pressing our tongue to our palate. We do this three to nine times.

Our tongue rules both our heart and the tendons of our body. This exercise helps to strengthen this connection, as well as tone our arms and open their meridians of which two are connected to our heart. Activating our heart meridians while moving sexual energy is a form of compassion alchemy. This exercise helps us to connect to the sensual energy of the earth. When we are in child pose, we make sure to relax with our tongue up.

REST (Repeat for yin chi cultivation).

DANCING DOLPHIN

We start by resting face down on our belly with our hands under our forehead. Then we inhale and lift our legs off the floor while squeezing our yoni tightly and pointing our feet. We lightly press down with our hand so that our neck (still lengthened and straight) slightly lifts off the floor (see fig. 9.15). Exhaling, we relax back down. We do this three to nine times.

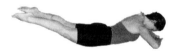
Fig. 9.15
Dancing dolphin

This exercise tightens our yoni while both opening the meridian of our legs and activating our spine. Making sure our tongue is up throughout the entire exercise, we can add rapid-yoni pulsing as we inhale and, unlike the other exercises, squeeze firmly on our exhale, relaxing our body back down to a neutral position.

REST (Repeat for yin chi cultivation).

FLYING GODDESS

This exercise is similar to the dolphin only this time we straighten our arms out in front of us with our hands in fists. As we inhale, we lift both our legs and arms off the floor and firmly grip our Jade Egg (see fig. 9.16). Exhale and relax back down to the neutral position. Rest for a moment and repeat three to nine times.

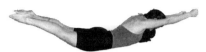

Fig. 9.16
Flying goddess

This exercise activates both our leg and arm meridians as well as our spine, thus integrating our entire body. Making sure we feel like we are initiating from our yoni, we may choose to pulse our yoni with our exhale. We may totally relax or we may choose to alternate between pulsing and relaxing. We can experiment with this one, keeping our tongue connected to our palate the whole time.

REST (Repeat for yin chi cultivation).

THE ART OF SCREWING AT ITS FINEST

OPENING THE QUA/GROIN

Beginning with our knees apart and our feet together (they do not need to be touching), we bend our arms so that we are holding some of our weight in our forearms. We inhale and dig into the floor with our hands as we pull our pelvis forward (see fig. 9.17). Then we exhale and push our palms into the floor as we push our pelvis back over our heels (see fig. 9.18).

This can be a very luscious experience. We may want to place some cushions under our knees for comfort. This exercise will really help to open our groin and the meridians that pass through this area. It will also allow us to absorb the sensual earth chi through our hands, enabling us to push it into our body for nurturing and enhancing our pleasure.

REST (Repeat for yin chi cultivation).

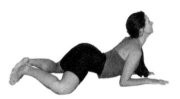

Fig. 9.17
Opening the qua/groin
while inhaling forward

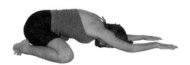

Fig. 9.18
Opening the qua/groin
while exhaling back

RECLAIM THE SCREW

In the same position as the previous exercise, we bring our elbows in a little so that we are able to sit back on our haunches. Now we gently start to move only our sacrum/tailbone in tiny spirals or screws. Keeping our spine straight and our bellies engaged will prevent back injury. We can also reverse the spiral or screw.

The screwing or spiraling of the sacrum is a fine art and is essential for practicing the higher arts of sexual alchemy. Keeping our tongue up helps as this exercise can initiate orgasm. We allow the sweet, sensual energy to spiral into and up our spine, breathing slowly and fully. Moaning can enhance our experience as can pulsing our tailbone down and up very slightly. As we breathe the chi up our spine and circulate it, we make sure that we do not move our hips. Only our sacrum. Isolating our sacrum is an important part of sexual practice as the more mobile our sacrum is, the more potent it becomes as a pump to move our sexual chi up our spine.

REST (Repeat for yin chi cultivation).

RECLAIM THE SCREW FOR TWO

The screw or the sacred spiral is another exercise that we can practice with our partner. Practicing this very subtle screwing and deep breathing is great when we feel like resting from the active part of sexual union. Remembering to circulate the chi that is generated through our orbits enhances both our connection and personal experience.

The smaller our physical movement, the bigger our chi movement. The reverse is also true—the bigger our physical movement, the smaller our chi movement.

REST (Repeat for yin chi cultivation).

After practicing any or all of the Jade Egg practices, we are bound to feel more energetic, whole, and alive. These practices are known to make us younger, stronger, more supple and open, as well as more orgasmic. It is important we enjoy our journey as we dive deeply into these ancient practices. Going slowly may not yield huge results right away; however, we will progress at our own natural pace, giving our body-mind-spirit the necessary time to integrate, assimilate and digest all the refined sexual energy. Once we master and feel comfortable with these core Jade Egg practices, we can move onto the more advanced practices which are done both seated and standing.

Were you able to establish a connection between your heart and your genitals?

How did it feel to train your body to invite rather than to be "pushed into"?

Which of the pelvic floor muscles were you able to begin to distinguish?

How has the activation of these muscles contributed to your sexual health and pleasure?

CHAPTER TEN

The Advanced Jade Egg Practices

Seated and Standing Practices of the Jade Egg

Let me take your hand
And look deep into your eyes
Let me just be there
Allowing you to be seen
Without agendas or judgments
Let me love fully
Accepting every little inch of you
So you may realize the truth within yourself
For me to be with you
Is an act of the Divine knowing itself
Peering at itself with itself
Touching itself with itself
Divine merging with Divine
This is the only way it can be
This is the yearning we all feel

CHAPTER GUIDE

N OW THAT WE HAVE BECOME COMFORTABLE using the Jade Egg as a core practice for enhancing our sensual and sexual lives, we are ready to expand our connection to our sensual selves by deepening our practice. Learning to move our energy when we are seated or standing brings a practical daily application to our sexual energy exercises.

How to Use This Portion of the Book

As with the previous Jade Egg practices, the advanced seated and standing practices are also designed to be experienced slowly and thoroughly, and either individually or as a continuous flow (moving from the lying down practices to the seated and standing practices). I have also placed a friendly reminder after each exercise to do both our compassion training and our yin or resting practice.

When we are first starting to do our seated practices, it is better to have our feet rooted into the Earth, rather than having our perineum touching the floor. If we do sit with our perineum on the floor, we may absorb too much unrefined Earth chi which may be too much for our body to digest and result in discomfort in the pelvis and lower back area. We may use our own discretion, however, and proceed with awareness.

As we practice, these exercises will bring us deeper into healing and cleansing our sexual centers and further refine our sensitivity so that we can become more and more aware of our omni-orgasmic energy.

JADE EGG PRACTICES: SEATED

CLEANSING OUR YONI

This exercise is a transitional exercise to help us move from our floor exercises into our seated exercises.

We begin this "cleansing the yoni" practice by sitting on our haunches or, alternately, placing a pillow or cushion under our pelvis. Using our hands as scoops, we make a scooping motion outside of our yoni while inhaling and imagining that we are scooping up any and all things that we no longer wish to have in our yoni. On our exhale, we turn our torso to one side and exhale a strong *Hah!* as we fall forward. When our hands hit the Earth/floor, we imagine discharging the negative or stagnant chi from our hands. Inhaling, we pull our hands along the Earth, drawing its pure, clean, healing energy up into our yoni (see fig. 10.1, next page). We

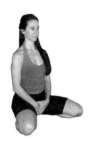

Fig 10.1
Cleansing our yoni
Inhale

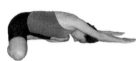

Fig 10.2
Cleansing our yoni
Exhale

release the same way, now on the other side, exhaling *Hah!* (see fig. 10.2). We can do as many as we feel are necessary to fully cleanse our yoni.

*This exercise cleans our yoni's subtle energies and replenishes her with fresh chi from the Earth. It also puts us more in touch with the Earth. As sensual women it is important that we love and honor mother Earth as she, like us, is also a succulent goddess and nurturing mother. In fact, this exercise is more powerful when done outdoors, right on the Earth herself. Releasing the **Hah** or **Pah** sound is also very clearing/cleansing.*

CUM-PASSION (Repeat to cultivate more compassion chi).

REST (Repeat for yin chi cultivation).

EGG-STATIC (ECSTATIC) PLAY

The following exercises are a repeat of our lying down Jade Egg practices; however, we now can do them either seated in a chair (which will allow our feet to root into Mother Earth) or seated on a meditation cushion (which will allow the perineum to root into Mother Earth).

SIPPING

To deepen our proficiency with sipping in our Jade Egg, we now perform all the sipping exercises from Chapter 9 (see pages 143-144), but this time from a seated position. When we sit up, we now have the extra challenge of gravity which can make the sipping exercises more difficult.

CUM-PASSION (Repeat to cultivate more compassion chi).

REST (Repeat for yin chi cultivation).

5-BUTTONS

Like our seated sipping exercises above, we now repeat all of the 5-button exercises (clitoris, anus, left and right transverse, and center, from Chapter 9, pages 148-152) in a seated position. This is a great way to practice these isolations. We can practice these exercises anywhere, even in our car or at the office!

CUM-PASSION (Repeat to cultivate more compassion chi).

REST (Repeat for yin chi cultivation).

SPIRAL DANCE

We can do the previous screwing techniques (see pages 156-157) while seated. Becoming aware of our tailbone/sacrum we gently make tiny spiral movements in both directions, remembering to keep our tongue up.

This exercise can be very stimulating, so circulating our sexual chi through our orbit during this exercise is helpful. This spiral dance is especially fantastic when performed when we are sitting on top of our partner. The smaller our spiral/screw, the more chi will build and move. Eventually, we can practice just moving our chi in a spiral without using any physical movement at all. This can be even more powerful. However, we keep practicing on the physical level until we feel confident that we can feel the chi moving in our body.

CUM-PASSION (Repeat to cultivate more compassion chi).

REST (Repeat for yin chi cultivation).

New Advanced Practices

The following advanced Jade Egg practices are unique to our seating practice.

SELF-HUGGING

Sitting with our ankles crossed and our knees pulled in close to our chest with our arms hugging our knees, we inhale and squeeze every muscle (especially our yoni) as much as we can while pulling our knees into our chest. As we exhale, we relax completely, letting our head drop and our spine sink so that our back is slouched into a C-shape. We repeat this practice as often as we like.

This exercise is very activating and we may feel orgasmic ripples or just strong currents of chi flowing through our body. This practice helps train our breath and body connection and helps us to understand the dynamics behind pleasure or the "tension and release" that occurs during a traditional orgasm. This exercise also trains us to perform dynamic tension with deep breathing that helps us to flush toxins out of our muscles.

CUM-PASSION (Repeat to cultivate more compassion chi).

REST (Repeat for yin chi cultivation).

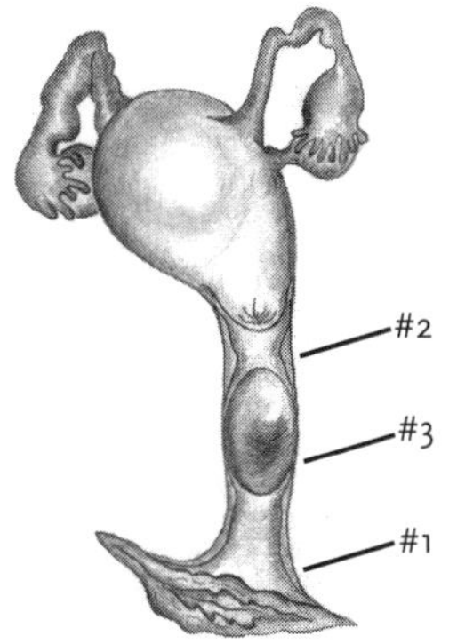

1-2-3 BLISS!

With this exercise, we separate our yoni into three parts: *bottom*, *top* and *middle*. Beginning at the bottom of our yoni (see #1 on fig. 10.3), we inhale and squeeze this part of our vagina, then we exhale and relax our vagina completely.

#2

#3

#1

Fig. 10.3
1-2-3 bliss!

Next, we move up to the top of our yoni (see #2 on fig. 10.3 on page 165) and again, we inhale-squeeze and exhale-relax. Finally, we go to the middle of our yoni (see #3 on fig. 10.3 on page 165), most likely where the egg is resting, and we inhale-squeeze, then exhale-relax. We repeat this exercise three to nine times.

This exercise helps to separate our yoni into three parts. It exercises the rings of muscle that surround our vaginal canal and enhances the movement of our chi to different parts of our body. An added bonus to this exercise is that it develops strong, dexterous yoni muscles allowing us to play any internally-placed item (finger, vajra, etc.) like a flute, which enhances our ability to pleasure ourselves without using our hands.

HELPFUL TIP: Using our hands can help us to create a mind-body connection. When we squeeze our yoni we bring our hands in towards each other, and when we relax, we move our hands apart. This movement also creates a visual image, allowing our mind to easily visualize what is happening internally.

ALTERNATE EXERCISE: Squeeze both zone #1 and zone #2 together at the same time (see fig. 10.4), then relax and squeeze zone #3. Inhale-squeeze #1 and #2, exhale-squeeze #3.

Another priceless technique is using our own finger internally during this exercise. This will give us direct feedback such as whether or not we are actually squeezing each section of our vagina, which section needs more practice, and which one needs more relaxation. Asking our partner during intercourse to give us loving feedback can create a playful atmosphere of fun and learning.

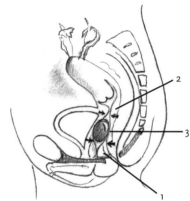

Fig. 10.4
Squeezing zone #1, #2 and #3

CUM-PASSION (Repeat to cultivate more compassion chi).

REST (Repeat for yin chi cultivation).

GRAB AND DANCE

Grabbing the egg with our vaginal muscles we move it up and down while keeping our hold on the egg, breathing slowly and deeply from our belly as we do this (see fig 10.5 on next page). To deepen our awareness and relaxation we softly smile inwardly.

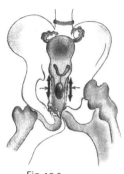

Fig. 10.5
Grab and dance

This is an excellent way of massaging our yoni as well as our egg, a finger or a vajra. It is a very grounding and energizing exercise as it activates both the spleen and liver systems in the body (see Chapter 8, for more on sexual reflexology). This is an ideal exercise for strengthening our yoni. In the traditional **yabyum** (tantra) position, this exercise and the 1-2-3 Bliss! exercise may be used to keep our partner's vajra firm and alert.

CUM-PASSION (Repeat to cultivate more compassion chi).

REST (Repeat for yin chi cultivation).

ENHANCING AMBROSIA: FEMALE EJACULATION

From our seated position, preferably on the floor, we inhale and sip our egg in and up. Exhaling we push down, moving our egg down (but not out). We really pull up and *really* push down as we exhale, relaxing as much as possible as we push down. We do this three to nine times.

This exercise may tire our muscles easily, so we do not want to do too many at first. Adding moaning and deep breathing will also enhance our sensations. We can also try using our finger to feel what is happening inside. If we rub along the urethral sponge (see page 219 for anatomy) as we do this exercise, we may induce a release of ambrosia (or ejaculate) (for more information on ambrosia, see Chapter 12). If we feel like urinating, we can bypass that feeling simply by relaxing into that feeling and keeping our breathing deep, while moaning and massaging firmly. If we don't release ambrosia, we do not have to worry about it as the delight from this exercise comes from being with ourselves, not just from the release. The point is more for us to exercise our yoni and have fun while doing so. It helps if we remember to stay connected to our heart, smile, and circulate our orgasmic chi.

CUM-PASSION (Repeat to cultivate more compassion chi).

REST (Repeat for yin chi cultivation).

STRING EVENTS

The following exercises require having a string or floss threaded through our Jade Egg. If we do not have an egg or are choosing not to use one at this time, we can still do the exercises simply by imagining a string instead. These exercises may be performed seated or reclining back on the bed or floor.

TUG OF LOVE

From a seated position, we lean back slightly and allow our pelvis to rock freely during this exercise. As we inhale, we pull down and away on the string while simultaneously sucking up hard on our egg internally. As we exhale, we just relax both our yoni and our hand that is pulling the string (see fig. 10.6). We do this three to nine times.

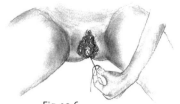

Fig. 10.6
Tug of love
Holding the string

This exercise increases the suction power of our yoni and our cervix. We only do as much as we feel is necessary. We may experience cramping in this exercise, so it is important to stop if we feel any discomfort and massage not only our belly, but around our yoni too. We can enhance our experience by being playful and gentle.

CUM-PASSION (Repeat to cultivate more compassion chi).

REST (Repeat for yin chi cultivation).

TUG OF LOVE ENHANCED

This time we inhale three sips (small breaths) as we suck up on our egg three times. As we exhale, we press and push our egg down, keeping a hold of the string as we do this. We do this exercise three to nine times.

This is another great exercise for increasing our suction power. Again, we only want to do as much as is comfortable for us, more is not always better. As we hold the string, we feel it pull and tighten as we suck up and we feel it loosen as we push down and out.

CUM-PASSION (Repeat to cultivate more compassion chi).

REST (Repeat for yin chi cultivation).

ADVANCED TUG OF LOVE

This exercise is a combination of a few movements and is done only once we are comfortable with the first two tug of love exercises. We begin by inhaling as we suck our egg in and exhaling as we push our egg out. Once we find a rhythm, we play with our egg while holding the string. Next, we apply tension very gently to our egg by pulling slightly on the string. We make sure we keep our egg inside and work our yoni muscles around our egg. In other words, we give our egg a massage by moving our pelvis a little in small spirals and tiny thrusts. Finally, we just let ourselves make love with our egg, letting ourselves dance while maintaining a constant pull on the string.

This can be an incredibly sweet and arousing technique as we let ourselves go and just dance with our egg. With this exercise, we can now start to integrate the natural movement of lovemaking into our Jade Egg practice.

CUM-PASSION (Repeat to cultivate more compassion chi).

REST (Repeat for yin chi cultivation).

STRUMMING FOR BLISS

Holding onto our egg's string while we rest our hand on our thigh, we start to vibrate our hand and thus the string. We do this while grabbing and holding our egg with our yoni, remembering to inhale and exhale slowly. *This exercise sends a vibration into our yoni via the string and egg, activating our different reflexology zones. As we start to feel our energy moving, we direct it through our orbit with our smile and intention, pausing occasionally to let our body awaken to this titillating sensation.*

CUM-PASSION (Repeat to cultivate more compassion chi).

REST (Repeat for yin chi cultivation).

STRUMMING FOR BLISS 2

This exercise is the same as the one above only this time we add the use of the left and right sides of our vagina, then the front and back of our vagina. We can also add the pelvic tilt and/or pelvic rocking technique, playing with the different ways of moving our pelvis while still sending a vibration into our yoni via the string and egg.

This exercise may be highly arousing. If so, we can simply enjoy and circulate our chi. This exercise will also teach us how to become very sensitive to our chi vibration and how to redirect it into the rest of our body for a fuller experience of bliss.

CUM-PASSION (Repeat to cultivate more compassion chi).

REST (Repeat for yin chi cultivation).

ADVANCED EROTIC STRING

For this exercise, we lie on our belly and rest the hand that is holding the string against our clitoris. We gently practice holding the string in our hand while sucking on our egg in order to keep it inside. Now we add some pelvic movements to enhance this suction tug-o-love experience. We may also want to add some moaning to open our throat center.

*This exercise is extremely arousing and generates a lot of chi as both our G-spot/**G-crest** area and our clitoris become activated. Making sure we keep our tongue up, we continuously move our aroused chi up into our orbit and cir-*

culate it. Lying on the floor may cause some discomfort in our hand that is underneath our pubic bone, so I recommend doing this exercise on a mat or bed. Also, if we are using floss, this exercise may break it, so being aware of this when doing this practice will ensure we are not taken by surprise.

CUM-PASSION (Repeat to cultivate more compassion chi).

REST (Repeat for yin chi cultivation).

SQUATTING FOR ECSTASY

The following exercises are advanced practices. If we try them and cannot do them, we must not be discouraged. We can simply smile love into ourselves and do other practices. Eventually we will build our strength to be able to do these exercises. Olympic athletes did not get where they are in a day, a week, or even a month! Becoming well versed in the higher sexual arts takes practice, time and *most* of all, enthusiasm, joy, compassion, and plenty of laughter.

ECSTATIC SQUAT

Squatting down as much as we can without feeling any discomfort, we now squeeze and relax our yoni in this posture. We can also move and stretch our spine a little while squatting (see fig. 10.7).

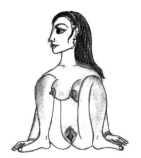

Fig. 10.7
Ecstatic squat

Squatting daily not only strengthens our legs, but it also opens up our qua/groin, helps our digestive system to have healthier elimination, helps us to release tensions that cause lower back pain, and increases the chi circulation in our leg meridians. Why is this important? These meridians bring chi to our sexual organs and if we have any energetic blocks in our groin, they can inhibit our sexual function. In North America, most of the activities we do promote a tight groin. For instance, if we spend more than an hour per day sitting in a chair, we may very likely have a tight groin. However, most of us are so accustomed to feeling this that we do not think of it as being bad. Tight groins often result in or are accompanied by a tight sacrum and sore lower back. Squatting regularly helps us to strengthen our thighs so that when we are in the on-top position, we can dance with much more power and freedom than before. Combining squatting with our yoni activation is key for allowing us to have the stamina for our on-top lovemaking.

CUM-PASSION (Repeat to cultivate more compassion chi).

REST (Repeat for yin chi cultivation).

ADVANCED SQUATTING

In the squatting position, we squeeze our yoni and internal pelvic muscles to lift us up and down. When we practice these squatting exercises, we can choose to partially support our weight by placing our hands on a chair or, in the case of **dual cultivation**, our partner can bend their arms at a right angle so we can hold onto their hands. We do this exercise using the breathing sequence of inhale, squeeze, lift, and exhale, relax, down. Now continuing with this movement we add:

1) Forward and back thrusts (tilting of the sacrum): Inhale, squeeze, forward lift; exhale, relax, down and back.

2) Forward and back thrusts with pulsing: Inhale, squeeze and pulse (squeezing quickly several times), forward lift; exhale, relax, down and back.

3) Side-to-side dance: Inhale, squeeze while lifting our left hip up; exhale relax down to center. Inhale and squeeze while lifting our right hip up; exhale and relax down to center. Each time we inhale, squeeze and lift one hip up slightly. This activates the corresponding side of our yoni.

4) Luscious circles: Inhale, squeeze, lift and make a full circle with either just our sacrum or our entire hip area (both create different sensations); exhale, relax back down. Circle in both directions.

5) Circle/snap: Inhale and relax (the opposite of what we have been doing in the other exercises) while we circle our hips; exhale and snap our hips forward. Snapping means we squeeze our yoni hard while thrusting our pelvis forward. Circle in both directions.

6) Sexy spirals: Inhale, squeeze and make very quick spirals while moving upwards; exhale and relaxing while spiraling back down (move up and down while spiraling). Circle in both directions.

7) Finally, we combine all of the above exercises as creatively as we desire for a powerful yoni dance.

All of these exercises will enable us to access the full range of our yoni (all its reflexology zones). These powerful practices create as much pleasure for us as they do for our partner. They also greatly enhance our ability to pleasure ourselves during intercourse and enable us to produce vaginal and uterine orgasms (versus only clitoral orgasms).

CUM-PASSION (Repeat to cultivate more compassion chi).

REST (Repeat for yin chi cultivation).

ALTERNATE POSITIONS FOR THE SQUATTING EXERCISES

Instead of squatting, we can kneel or partially kneel (with one leg kneeling, one leg squatting), making sure we have sufficient padding under our knees.

This will work out our thighs, so we must not do this modification if we have sore knees or feel any pain in our joints.

CUM-PASSION (Repeat to cultivate more compassion chi).

REST (Repeat for yin chi cultivation).

JADE EGG PRACTICES: STANDING

TIPS FOR STANDING PRACTICE

When we practice standing we must be prepared to have much more gravity to contend with. While standing, some of us may find that our natural tendency is to *push* down with our pelvic muscles. However, by doing so, we sometimes find that we inadvertently push our egg out. Beginning our standing practice with our legs close together and our feet pointed inwards facilitates holding in our egg. Once our muscles are trained to hold our egg, then we are able to do the exercises while standing with our feet parallel and apart. The most advanced standing posture is with our feet hip-width apart or wider in the horse stance position (see fig. 10.8). Some days, we may feel the need to turn our feet inward (which helps to close our yoni) while on other days, the wide stance may feel perfectly fine. As with all the practices, it is important that we remain non-judgmental about our progress and that we keep in mind that wherever our body is at today, is perfect.

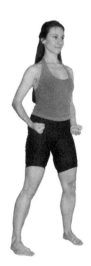

Fig. 10.8
Horse stance

STANDING THRUSTS AND SPIRALS

STANDING THRUSTS

Standing in whichever position works best for us, we begin to move our sacrum forward and back. First, we move just our tailbone, then we eventually work up to moving our entire pelvis. Our breath sequence goes like this: inhale, squeeze forward; exhale, relax back.

When we are standing, we must make sure that we do not fully let go of our egg (even when we relax) as it might come out. Instead, we smile (this slightly engages our perineum) and become aware that we are gently holding onto our egg when we are relaxing. We keep our tongue up to circulate our energy.

CUM-PASSION (Repeat to cultivate more compassion chi).

REST (Repeat for yin chi cultivation).

STANDING SPIRALS

Beginning with tiny spirals of our tailbone, we eventually work up to circling our entire pelvis. We do this in both directions, coordinating our movement with our breath and imagining that there is a weight attached to our tailbone or our Jade Egg.

If we pay attention inwardly, we will find that this exercise creates a strong upward flow of aroused chi. Keeping our tongue up and smiling encourages our chi to move through our micro-cosmic orbit.

CUM-PASSION (Repeat to cultivate more compassion chi).

REST (Repeat for yin chi cultivation).

NO HAND CLAPPING

For this exercise, we squeeze our vaginal muscles, becoming aware of the entire left side of our yoni and the entire right side of our yoni pressing (or moving) towards each other. Then we relax. We continue this practice of inhaling and feeling the right and left sides of our yoni come together or *clap* (see fig. 10.9). Then we exhale and relax. Sometimes it is useful to create a mind-body connection by moving our hands to depict what is occurring internally. If we choose to do this, we simply bring our hands in front of our genitals and as we squeeze and clap our vagina, we bring our hands towards each other

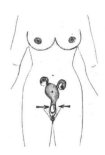

Fig. 10.9
Right and left
No hand clapping

in a silent *clap.* As we relax, we then move our hands away from each other. We do this exercise three to nine time's and imagine our yoni clapping.

This exercise strengthens our yoni and activates our thrusting channels. If we remain aware of the left and right sides of the body as we do this, we may be able to sense the chi moving through our thrusting channels.

CUM-PASSION (Repeat to cultivate more compassion chi).

REST (Repeat for yin chi cultivation).

FRONT TO BACK CLAPPING

This exercise is the same as the one above only now we are using the front and back pelvic muscles. It is easier if we actually place one hand over our womb in the front near the pubic bone, and the other on our sacrum (with our finger tips on our tailbone). Now, we press our hands into our body and feel how this helps us connect with our internal muscles that are also moving towards each other. Our breathing sequence is inhale and press; exhale and relax. Even though our hands are moving in a clapping motion externally, we may feel as though the movement is originating internally through our front and back pelvic muscles (see fig. 10.10).

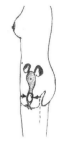

Fig. 10.10
Front and back
No hand clapping

During this practice, our vagina and rectum may feel like they are pressing in towards and out away from each other. This is highly activating for the front and back channels of our micro-cosmic orbit. Relaxing as fully as possible when we do this one, we do not use any force for the clapping. We simply smile, relax and feel.

CUM-PASSION (Repeat to cultivate more compassion chi).

REST (Repeat for yin chi cultivation).

UP AND DOWN CLAPPING

Now we imagine the top of our yoni (the cervix itself) and the bottom of our yoni (the inner lips and opening) coming together and moving apart. Inhale and press the top and bottom together; exhale and relax, and repeat three to nine times.

During this exercise, our vaginal canal will feel as though it is getting shorter and longer. Practicing this is important because it allows us to eventually work with two Jade Eggs at once and/or create stronger suction power in our yoni.

CUM-PASSION (Repeat to cultivate more compassion chi).

REST (Repeat for yin chi cultivation).

ADDITIONAL STANDING PRACTICES

STANDING SUCTION

In this practice, we pull up our egg using three short inhales, then we push down our egg using three short exhales. Inhale up-up-up and exhale down-down-down. This is done three to nine times.

This exercise is potentially very arousing. It works out our cervix and the upper area of our yoni (although we also feel the rest of our yoni working). We can sense our chi rise as we inhale and circulate as we exhale. Using a tiny bit of muscular force, we can focus more on our chi/breath when pushing down to make sure we don't push our egg all the way out.

CUM-PASSION (Repeat to cultivate more compassion chi).

REST (Repeat for yin chi cultivation).

GOOD VIBRATIONS

Tightening our yoni as much as possible, we rock our pelvis forward. We keep tightening (holding on to the tension) as we gently force our pelvis to rock backwards, sticking our tailbone up. If we do this correctly, we will feel a quick vibration of our pelvis as we move and press it back. This vibration is a result of our muscle tension: we experience a similar feeling when we tighten our bicep and maintain tension as we straighten our arm. Our breath sequence for this practice is inhale and tighten forward; exhale and tighten back. Again, we do this three to nine times.

This exercise is very sensual as the tiny vibrations wake-up our pelvis and spine. We can also do this seated. Relaxing afterwards aids us to let go of all our muscular tension. If we feel sore, we can stop and massage our whole pelvic area.

CUM-PASSION (Repeat to cultivate more compassion chi).

REST (Repeat for yin chi cultivation).

GOOD VIBRATIONS ADVANCED

This is the same exercise as the previous one except we add some new pelvic movements. This time, we move side-to-side and diagonally while keeping the same breath pattern: inhale, squeeze hard, and move in one direction; exhale, keep squeezing, and move in the opposite direction.

This exercise brings the vibration sensation into all parts of our pelvis. We can get creative with this one if we enjoy it and we can also try this with our partner inside of us.

CUM-PASSION (Repeat to cultivate more compassion chi).

REST (Repeat for yin chi cultivation).

SACRED SHIMMY

We begin by shimmying. If we do not have experience with producing a shimmy, we can simply relax our knees and start moving them back and forth quickly. This knee movement will affect our pelvis, making it jiggle or shimmy. With practice, our shimmy will start in our pelvis, rather than our knees. As we do our own version of a shimmy, we will feel the vibration in our pelvis and let the sensation expand into the rest of our body. Playing with this shimmy energy invigorates every cell in our body with vital life force.

This exercise is taken from belly dancing, which is an excellent exercise for maintaining both our pelvic health and the spontaneous joy that comes from expressing energy through the movement of our body. Relaxation is key to a successful shimmy.

CUM-PASSION (Repeat to cultivate more compassion chi).

REST (Repeat for yin chi cultivation).

Ending Our Jade Egg Practice

We can end our Jade Egg practice at any point. However, we must always remember to collect the energy/chi that is generated throughout our practice and store it in our navel (tan tien), then deeply rest in yin. The storing is very important as it ensures that we are centered after doing our expanding and energy heightening sexual practices. Also, storing our chi is vital to rejuvenating our body. If we do not practice storing our chi, then most of the efforts of our sexual practice is lost. The yin rest ensures we absorb, integrate, and assimilate all the vitality and healing from our sexual practice.

Storing the Chi

Taking a moment to sense all the chi that has built up in our practice, we smile down to our navel to begin collecting the chi. We imagine the chi spiraling three, nine, or thirty-six times counterclockwise. Then we visualize the spiral moving clockwise three, nine, or twenty-four times. We then form a beautiful pearl of refined sexual chi and place it in our cauldron to store it.

This invaluable practice enables us to access this refined creative energy at any time simply through smiling down at our navel and activating the stored pearl.

Yin Time

The longer we can rest and *do nothing* after our practice, the better. If we only have one minute, then we rest for one minute. If we have more time, we rest longer. It is a time to practice the art of be-ing, a quality that is part of our feminine, receptive energy—open, willing and waiting. This form of yin practice cultivates the feminine aspect of ourselves more deeply.

Self Massage

After we rest, we can give ourselves a little chi shower by gently tapping our entire body from the top of our head to the bottom of our feet, and from the front to the back. If we have more time, we can massage our entire body from head to feet first, then follow this with the chi shower.

For the Rest of Our Day

For the rest of the day, let us keep smiling and keep our tongue up as often as we can, breathing deeply and slowly, and remembering to give our egg a little squeeze now and again (if we choose to wear it throughout the day). We may even want to sleep with our egg inside. Many of my students have reported experiencing more vivid dreams and more restful sleep when the egg is inside. For those of us who cannot yet hold our egg in, this night-time practice helps us to make progress since our yoni plays with our egg as we sleep.

If we do wear our egg throughout the day or at night, we must make sure we remember that it is still there when we go to the bathroom! Many of us sensual women have lost our eggs in the toilet; however, most of us were able to recover our egg and disinfect it.

More Subtle, Advanced Practices

Enhancing Our Advanced Practice with Eye Power

The iris of our eye is intricately linked to the sphincter muscles of our body. Using this connection, we can control our chi movement by subtly squeezing and moving our eyes. As we develop our skills, we also hone our ability to create powerful movements of chi without much physical movement. Our chi moves where our eyes look. To keep the chi inside of us, we close our eyes. To exchange our chi, we open our eyes and look at the person or at nature, or whomever/whatever we would like to exchange energy with. To move our chi up, we roll our eyes up. Similarly, to move our chi to the navel, we look at our navel. This practice requires a developed sensitivity that may come naturally for some of us, but may require more practice for others.

Eye Power

With any of the practices, we can create more subtle versions of them by using our eyes. To move our chi through our left and right thrusting channels, we can move our eyes (not our head) to look in the direction we desire to move our chi. Looking in our desired direction, we squint very lightly and gently (as if we are closing and opening the iris of each eye), this eye action results in the squeezing and releasing of our yoni, anus, and sphincter muscles.

This exercise generates and moves a lot of chi. You can apply this modification to most of the Jade Egg practices in both this and the previous chapter.

"I Can't Feel My Egg"

"I can't feel my egg!" is one of the most common complaints that come up during a Jade Egg seminar. As women, we often feel very concerned that something is wrong with us if we cannot feel our egg. In truth there is absolutely nothing wrong with us. In fact, our egg is not meant to be felt! Imagine feeling a tampon all the time—it could get quite annoying.

The purpose of the Jade Egg is not to create bone-shaking orgasms or other similar sensations (though they are possible). It is to help us develop our awareness, sensitivity, and dexterity. As sensual women, the more we develop our awareness about our yoni and our internal anatomy, the more we are able to perceive what has always been there: an infinite resource of bliss. This awareness leads to increased sensitivity. As we play with our egg, the tissues of our genitals become more and more sensitive and capable of expressing sensation. This increased sensation and dexterity, coupled with a developing awareness of our vagina, leads to our experience of heightened pleasure.

To an untrained nose, a wine will smell like any other, yet to a trained nose, each wine has a distinct bouquet of scents. This is true for any of our senses. The more they are developed and exercised, the more finely tuned they become. As we learn how to differentiate between the different muscles in our vagina and our pelvis, our awareness of our egg and the subtle (and sometimes not so subtle) sensations of its movements will increase.

If we cannot feel our egg, we must not worry as this is perfectly normal. By simply focusing on our breathing, our love of ourselves, and relaxing, our own awareness and sensitivity will develop and expand. If we play like a child, with wonderment and awe, we will forget what we think it should feel like and accept the invitation into our most mysterious and powerful expression with great delight.

> *Questions: Are you vaginally sensitive—that is, do you experience orgasm through vaginal stimulation? How does the idea of sensitizing your vagina inspire you to investigate the possibilities of the Jade Egg teachings?*

"I have pain after practicing"

Another common complaint I hear from women who are learning to use the Jade Egg is of pain in their genitals or pelvic region during or after the practice. The pain is normally described as a dull ache or cramping. The cause of this discomfort comes from the use of muscles that may have never been used before. Just like working out in a gym, we must go slowly and start with short, easy workouts to prevent injury or strain. The same goes for our Jade Egg exercises. The slower we go and the gentler we are, the more confidence we will start to build about our sexual and sensual capabilities while enhancing our sexual pleasure and health

If we do feel pain or discomfort during the exercises, we must stop, rest and massage our belly and genitals. Remembering to breathe slowly and deeply and to practice the techniques with as much inner awareness as possible also helps eliminate or prevent pain from occurring. It is good for us to rest between each exercise and to maintain an easy practice schedule at the beginning. If we experience severe or sharp pain, we must stop immediately and consult our doctor as our pain may be due to other factors that may require professional attention.

Growing Heart versus Growing Ego

This section is dedicated to those of us who choose to embark on our journey of sexual energy cultivation with the help of a live teacher. There are many teachers of sexual traditions in the world, but for all of them, one of the greatest challenges is to grow beyond their ego's desire for power. Engaging in sexual contact with a student is entirely unnecessary as all the teachings can be transmitted without actually having to physically touch another. All teachers in the field of sexual cultivation have the responsibility to uphold the highest degree of compassion and integrity when transmitting this information to their students. It is vital that we recognize that we may be charmed and mesmerized by the magnetism of people who do this practice and that we know the difference between a teacher who is there to help us master ourselves versus a teacher who is using us to grow their own ego and energy. The Jade Goddess teachings and the Art of Succulent Living philosophy are dedicated to empowering us women to emerge as our own masters, lovers, and guides so that we may exercise wisdom and discernment in all of our life choices.

> *Questions: How will you choose your teacher(s)? What standard of sexual education do you have?*

Possible Side Effect of These and Other Jade Egg Exercises

When I met Dr. Rachel Abrams (co-author of *The Multi-Orgasmic Woman*), she informed me that women who have long cervical necks (the neck of the uterus) tend to be more orgasmic than women with short cervical necks. We also noticed that women who practice frequently with the Jade Egg have longer cervical necks. More research is still needed on this topic; however, it is interesting to note that these Jade Egg exercises may change our physiology so we become more and more orgasmic.

Additional Effects of Aroused Sexual Practice

These more advanced practices are considered hot practices. Hot practice is a term used to describe exercises that cultivates aroused sexual energy, whereas cool practice cultivates un-aroused sexual energy. Most of the Jade Egg practices and sexual qi gong are considered to be cool practice since they cultivate un-aroused sexual energy. Hot practice is usually not taught by most Tao instructors due to its erotic nature and to the comfort levels of both the instructor and the students. This label is misleading since un-aroused energy for women tends to feel hot or warm, while aroused energy tends to feel cool. When we orgasm and feel the need to be covered due to feeling cold, that is a concrete example of this cool energy. Using the upward draw technique is recommended (see Chapter 8) in cases of aroused practice. This will help to move the aroused energy up into the brain and nurture our master glands.

When we cannot reach orgasm from vaginal penetration this is often because we are not able to fully relax into our pleasure while trusting penetration. We also may not have activated our clitoral system by using our vaginal dexterity, strength and suppleness. These exercises will enhance our ability to access our clitoral system by increasing our awareness and strength of our pelvic floor muscles. These exercises also help us to build our self-confidence along with our ability to relax while building up our sexual excitement and energy. The more we keep our tongue up, breathe from our belly, and activate our throat through moaning, the more we will activate our sex center.

As we do more advanced practices, we begin to learn how our sexual energy can be very subtle and refined. We also embrace the added challenge of gravity and of handling more and more aroused sexual chi with greater and greater mastery. Deepening our connection to our body through using the Jade Egg, we begin desiring to care for our yoni and our breasts in a much more loving, conscious and sacred way. Let us now move into caring for both our yoni and breasts.

Were you able to sense your internal energy more during the egg practice?

What emotions did you feel during the exercises?

How has this practice affected your sexual energy?

CHAPTER ELEVEN

Yoni and Breast Care

Nurturing and Caring for
Our Sensual Selves

My breast
full and firm
erect attention draws
up the juice
sweet, golden honey dew
dripping
as it seeks the circular
path to the peak
round and round and round
Oh yes
the earthquakes and sighs
as the sun covers
her in his
golden warmth
again and again
Goddess greets God

CHAPTER GUIDE

Now that we have explored our abilities with the Jade Egg, we now have a solid understanding of the power and dexterity of our yoni. This invites us to investigate a new topic: the many options we have for caring for the health of our genitals. Equally, our breasts play a big role in balancing and enhancing our sexual energy and hormones. Thus, as emerging sensual women, we must begin to nurture and care for these precious parts of our body with greater dedication. In this chapter, we will explore the side of the Art of Succulent Living and the Jade Goddess teachings that include the rich process of caring for both our yoni and our breasts while cultivating our awareness of their interconnection.

How to Use This Portion of the Book

This portion of the book contains two sections. The first section is dedicated to the care of our yoni (our sexual center). The second section is dedicated to caring for our breasts (our love center). This chapter blends philosophy with practicality, inspiring us to seek new and healthy ways to care for our sacred body. Reading it in its entirety prior to doing any of the suggested practices is recommended as an initial orientation to the material. However, the information in this chapter can stand on its own or be read at any point during our exploration of the Jade Goddess teachings. Some of the exercises here may stretch our boundaries of personal comfort. Therefore, it may help us to remember that everything is simply offered as an invitation, not as a command. After our first read through, we can then use the Yoni and Breast Care chapter guide to select where we would like to begin our self-nurturing practice. As sensual women, we can access much wisdom through balancing and nurturing our two sacred centers (our sexual center and our love center) both individually and simultaneously.

What is a Yoni?

"When watered with love, this magical flower blossoms into a portal that invites us back into Source." — DJ

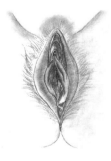

The first section of this chapter is dedicated to our yoni care. The word *yoni* is a Sanskrit word meaning womb or female genitalia. It is the preferred word within the Jade Goddess teachings as it describes of our genitals as being a sacred place or temple. As sensual women, we understand our yoni to be the seat of our power. It is the center where our creative life force is expressed, either in the creation of a child or in recreating ourselves as sensual women. Our creative life force is also known as our vital life force or sexual energy, and it is the essential ingredient in our creative process.

By exploring the concept of honoring and caring for our yoni, we will feel a renewed reverence for the creative source within us. In everyday life, our yoni may experience lack of or infrequent touch. She may be powdered or plugged up with unnatural scents or be asphyxiated by underwear that doesn't let her breathe. When we shift this unconscious behavior to one of honoring our yoni, we can begin to feel compassion and properly care for this part of us that is precious and beautiful.

> Questions: How do you treat your yoni? What is your relationship to this part of your body?

Knowing Our Yoni Is Our Power

Aside from never knowing what our own genitals look like, few of us are comfortable with the different scents and discharges released by our yoni throughout our cycle. One aspect of allowing sensuality to emerge involves accepting every little corner of our body, including our sexual organs. As sensual women, we take time to know ourselves intimately. We take the time to explore our entire body and use this exploration as a way to reclaim any loss of intimacy that may have occurred since the innocence of our childhood.

Every yoni is unique, just like the many different flowers of a garden. Getting to know our yoni is an essential part of reclaiming our power and succulence as women. The best way to get to know our yoni is to look at her. The number of us women who do not know what our genitals look like is staggering. Although looking at our genitals may seem intimidating or frightening, its importance is profound. It is the beginning of our journey of expanding both our pleasure and self-love as emerging sensual women.

Exercise: Reclaiming our yoni

By using a mirror, we can discover our yoni's unique beauty in a safe, sacred, unrushed manner. No matter what thoughts or feelings that arise for us, if we continue to breathe deeply, we can keep our hearts open and soft. Touching ourselves with loving curiosity, we can examine our labia (outer and inner lips, see fig. 11.1 on page 189). Spreading them open, we can then admire the sacred gate of our vaginal opening as well as our pearl of bliss (clitoris). Let's take our time and feel the love of our heart in our finger tips as we explore ourselves and discover the magnificence of our yoni. Resting afterwards and writing down in a journal any feeling or thoughts that may have come up for us during the experience, can provide us with wonderful insights. I fondly call this activity *yoni journaling*, where we write from the perspective of our yoni.

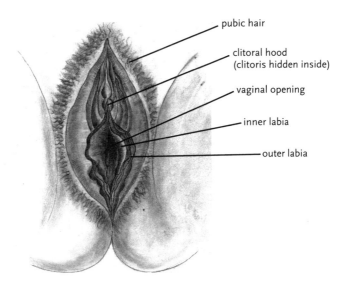

pubic hair

clitoral hood
(clitoris hidden inside)

vaginal opening

inner labia

outer labia

Fig. 11.1
Yoni anatomy

Questions: How does it feel to look at your yoni? What are the benefits of knowing your sexual anatomy visually? What insights do you find when you journal from your yoni's perspective?

Taste Test

In the secret teachings of the Jade Goddess all of our fluids produced by our body are considered sacred. Tears, saliva, sweat and sexual secretions all have different qualities of energy to offer us and as sensual women we accept our body as sacred and view our secretions as precious elixir. We then are able to taste and smell our yoni as a way of getting to understand her. This form of intimacy with ourselves has numerous benefits including the ability to monitor the health of our genitals. Quite often there is a change of smell and taste in our yoni when there is an imbalance or stress in our body. By using this method of self-analysis, a woman may diagnose and prevent imbalances from becoming problems. Daily monitoring through tasting and smelling the yoni's secretions deepens self-intimacy and trust in the ability to heal and truly know ourselves.

Exercise: A taste of wisdom

Using a clean finger, we gently enter our vaginal canal and relax in this position for a moment, feeling both with our vagina and our finger the sensations created by penetration. Then we slowly pull out our finger and smell and taste it, noticing our scent and opening our awareness to the flavor of our essence. Our smell and taste may change depending on a variety of factors such as where we are in our cycle, if we are hydrated or not, if we have eaten spicy foods, garlic, if we have used latex or any products other than our natural secretions during sexual activity, and whether or not our partner has ejaculated inside of us. After our taste test experience, we can rest and then write down our feelings and our experience in our yoni journal.

Questions: How does your yoni taste and smell? How do you feel about this taste and smell? Did you notice this taste and smell change over a period of time or after different life experiences?

Natural Aphrodisiac

Pheromones are very powerful aphrodisiacs. Most seductive perfumes contain some sort of pheromone that is attractive to others. The most natural and affordable source of pheromones a sensual woman can use is found in our own yoni. We can make use of this knowledge by using a little of our yoni essence on our body, applying it to where we typically apply our perfume: wrists, neck, under our breasts. With no noticeable odor, yet like the perfume from an exotic flower, our essence works its charm, inviting us to begin valuing our yoni essence as a highly potent aphrodisiac.

STORY: *Rekindling passion*

A woman who did not know how to seduce her husband (long-standing marriage) came to me looking for a solution. She reported that her husband rarely paid attention to her and rarely initiated sexual contact. I offered her the secret of the attractive power of her yoni's essence and instructed her to anoint her body with her own secretions. That evening, after she anointed herself, he not only noticed her, he suddenly became very attentive, and they enjoyed wonderful love making for the first time in a very long time.

Questions: Have you tried this exercise? What were the results?

Women With Moon Cycles

As women, we become very powerful during our moon cycle. During this period of time, we experience a tremendous increase in our ability to feel and sense (our psychic ability). We may feel overwhelmed if there is little or no understanding of this phenomenon. Our lack of understanding about this increase in our sensitivity may be partially responsible for creating some of our mood swings. These emotional imbalances are normally thought of as PMS symptoms in our Western society, yet remain virtually unheard of to women who live in close harmony with their body. When we as sensual women start to know ourselves, start eating a healthier diet, take the time to honor our feelings and our body, and practice staying connected to the natural energies around us, a lot of our mood-swings diminish or disappear entirely.

> Questions: Do you experience mood swings with your moon cycle? Do you believe PMS is natural?

As sensual women, we can use the Jade Goddess breast exercises and the ovarian breathing to reduce the volume of blood we lose with each moon (menstrual) cycle, as well as eliminating our painful PMS symptoms. This is the modern meaning of **Slaying the Red Dragon**, our ability to reduce or eliminate PMS symptoms. Learning and reclaiming the ability to affect change in our body is an integral part of practicing the Art of Succulent Living.

STORY: Transforming cramps into pleasure

A student of mine was a track runner who suffered tremendous cramps that caused her to use strong medication and to stay a few days in bed. After practicing with the Jade Egg and doing some of the sexual qi gong exercises I recommended, she was shocked to find that her next period was painless. She didn't need the prescription drugs, and she didn't need a few days in bed. In fact, she hardly noticed that she was having a moon-cycle at all. Her success was due to allowing her body to harmonize itself. A balanced body is a healthy body—this includes the health of one's sexual organs!

Feminine Products

As modern women we do not take the time to value the natural ebb and flow of energy that our moon cycles amplify, and we often desire a quick and simple solution to control this "messy" and "annoying" time. We use scented tampons, pads, and different pain medications as a means to ignore our moon blood and moon cycle. We are unaware (or ignore) that regular use of these commercial pads and tampons may possibly be a health hazard. These products contain various substances, one of which is rayon. Rayon is derived from wood and subjected to being bleached with chlorine. Hilary Kaplan of Yale University states, "Chlorine bleaching produces the chemical commonly known as dioxin, which is classified as a "known human carcinogen" by the International Agency for Research on Cancer, a branch of the World Health Organization." Research on this topic is insufficient, yet what is stated is that there are possible hazards with repeated exposure. Monthly use of these products is a significant repeated exposure; thus, we must investigate this topic more fully to satisfy our personal queries. Until the results indicate there is absolutely no hazard to our health, we women are wise to investigate natural moon care options.

Healthy Moon-Care Options

For a healthy yoni, it is best to use all natural products. Here is a list of some options:

* organic tampons
* cotton (re-useable) pads
* The Keeper (natural rubber)

The Keeper is my favorite option as it is made of natural rubber and is re-useable. It can be tricky to use at first, but with practice it is just as comfortable as a tampon. Use of the Keeper invites us to become familiar with our moon cycle as we can monitor the exact amount and quality of our blood and other fluids released within our moon cycle. One bonus of using the Keeper is that it creates no environmental waste and gives us the option to use our blood in our garden if we choose. Moon blood has long been used to fertilize gardens. We simply pour the contents of our Keeper into a watering can, then dilute it. We can then water our plants with its revitalizing essence.

If our moon time is not too heavy, then even just folding a piece of tissue in our underwear could be enough. Again, our sexual practices (breast massage, ovarian breathing and compression, the upward draw, and our Jade Egg practices) help to reduce our moon flow making our blood clear and healthy. Combining the practices with good diet will greatly reduce most of our sexual issues.

Moon-Time (Menstrual) Care

Culturally, there has been a movement away from honoring the feminine and, as a result, we have made our menstrual blood dirty, bad, wrong or "a problem". As sensual women, we reclaim the sacredness of our moon (menstrual) blood by understanding that nothing our body naturally produces is dirty, bad, wrong or "a problem". It only becomes that way when we attach negative beliefs to it. In the Jade Goddess teachings, these beliefs are examined and replaced with the understanding that our moon-time (menstrual period) is very sacred.

Questions: What are your current beliefs around menstruation? Do you view your blood as sacred or something annoying or dirty?

Exercise: Reconnecting to our moon cycle

Let's take a moment to write down all our beliefs around our moon cycle (menstrual cycle) and to notice how many of our beliefs/ideas are positive and how many are negative. Now let's replace our negative beliefs with new, life-affirming affirmations. Resting, let's notice how we feel with our new beliefs about our body as a woman.

Our Yoni and Our Diet

"We are what we eat" applies to all parts of our body including our genitals. Diet, proper digestion, and hydration all play a big role in the scent and flavor of our yoni. The quality of our yoni's secretions and odor is dependent on the nature of the food we consume. When we eat junk food or food that has a strong flavor such as garlic or other spices, our yoni will soon smell and taste of that same food. For example, pungent foods equal pungent odor, sour food equal sour taste, and so on. Eating a healthy diet with plenty of green vegetables and unprocessed food will enhance the pleasant smell of our yoni.

Colon health is another factor that plays a big part in our yoni's hygiene. Feces that is impacted in our colon is toxic to our body and leads to bad breath and strong scented yonis. Also, there is often a connection between spastic colons and spastic vagina's. If there is trauma in the colon, it can be felt in the genitals, and if there is trauma in the genitals, it can be felt in the colon. Many of us who suffer from these spasms will benefit from bringing our attention to cleansing our colon and facing the deeper issues that caused our imbalance in the first place. Taking care of our body as a living, sacred temple enhances the healing of all our tissues. There are many theories on colon cleansing, from herbs to enemas to colonics. As sensual women, we are wise to investigate our options and choose what methodology feels best for our healing.

If diet and clean colons are not an issue, most likely the hydration of our body is. Hydration plays a key role in our sexual health (and the health of our entire body). Proper hydration helps us to eliminate some unpleasant body and yoni odors, as well as provides our body with more *juiciness*. If we are older women suffering from vaginal dryness we may wish to investigate our level of hydration and the strength of our perineum. All women who release ambrosia are well aware of how important optimal hydration is for enhancing our experience.

> *Questions: What is your diet like? Have you noticed a relationship between the health of your colon and the smell of your yoni? Do you know if you are well-hydrated?*

Moisturized Yoni

As with any health regime, balance is our goal. An overly damp yoni may lead to internal imbalances, while an overly dry yoni can be painful and uncomfortable. Keeping our yoni clean, aired out, occasionally exposed to the sun, and by eating a healthy diet, honoring our emotions, and moisturizing our yoni leaves her vibrant, healthy and sweet.

The skin of our yoni, in general, tends to be quite sensitive and tender and requires special attention. Washing her with harsh soaps can be irritating and drying. Often when we women complain of dryness or soreness it is because we have over-washed our yoni with harsh soaps.

If our yoni is dry or irritated, we may want to investigate using a different soap. Trying a very gentle, natural and unscented soap and rinsing well afterwards may help. All skin, even our yoni skin, benefits from a good moisturizer that is something natural and non glycerin-based. Also, we can spritz our yoni with rose water, or add a bit of aloe vera gel or natural salve to our daily moisturizing care. These are all great ways to protect our yoni.

To moisturize our yoni, we place some oil or gel on our clean fingers and we gently massage the skin of our outer and inner labia. Doing this every morning as an anointing ritual is sensually enjoyable. Practicing the inner smiling to our yoni during the application further increases our relationship of love with and awareness of our yoni.

> *Question: What does your yoni feel like after using a gentler soap and moisturizer?*

Trim and Proper

The subject of our pubic hairs and their maintenance is a little more common in the 21st century. As sensual women we all are very unique in how we choose to coif our pubes. Some of us women like long hair, some of us like to be bald, and some of us like to be trimmed in a particular design. Aside from personal preference, caring for our pubic hairs has an impact on the hygiene of our yoni. If we have longer pubic hair, we need to wash it carefully so that the odor of urine does not imbue it. A common complaint from those who enjoy orally honoring yonis is that pubic hairs that smell strongly of urine is a turn-off. Keeping our pubic hairs trimmed or waxing them completely off also helps to eliminate the uric odor.

STORY: *Clear-cutting our bush*

Many years ago, I was at a beautiful clothing-optional lake, and stood nude on a dock in the sunshine. An older woman who was sunning her bald yoni eyeing my abundant bush, turned and asked me, "would you like to know a sexual secret?" "Of course!", I eagerly replied. Smiling, she offered the following: "If you trim your bush you will feel more. Trust me on this." I thought this was a little strange, yet a few months later I decided to try out this secret. Lo and behold, I was amazed at the sensation! I could barely handle the feeling of my underwear against my newly exposed skin. When my lover orally honored me that evening, I had the most amazing orgasms! I could feel so much more, even with penetration. It was as though the hair had been buffering or protecting this sacred place and removing it exposed ultra sensitive skin. To this day, I keep my hair trimmed and enjoy the enhanced feelings of pleasure. Just ask anyone who shaves their head how sensitive their scalp is and how pleasurable it is for them to have it massaged and touched.

Choosing our Pubic-Style

Trimming or styling our pubic hairs is not for all of us; however, it is good to know what our options are if we are considering to venture into the art of pubic hair maintenance. Below is a list of pubic hair care options:

SHAVING
Shaving with a razor requires daily maintenance as the *sharp* re-growth may get uncomfortable. This method is quick and reliable, yet can be itchy and uncomfortable if the hairs are allowed to grow in.

TRIMMING
Some of us use an electric trimmer to trim our hairs down to the length we enjoy. This is also very convenient and can at times cause us some itchiness depending on how short our hairs are trimmed.

Waxing choices range from a simple bikini wax (where the hairs that are left out when wearing a bikini bottom are removed) to a full Brazilian wax (where all the hair on our labia, etc., are removed). Waxing can be painful, and its best to have a professional do this. Some of us do it ourselves, but for first timers, I highly recommend going to someone who is very skilled. Use of a French wax is better for the genital hairs as it pulls the least on the skin and is a less painful choice. After repeated waxing our hairs may thin out, become softer, and grow in slower than after shaving and trimming. Waxing is painful, although the pain decreases with repeated sessions. However, there is also the possibility of ingrown hairs.

Note: Tweezing stray hairs is commonly done along with waxing. This is fine for a few hairs, but is labor intensive and a little painful.

LASER

This technique permanently reduces our hair and heals any in-grown scars. Laser is very expensive and can only be done at laser-certified centers. About four to five sessions are needed for a full reduction.

Ultimately, how we care for our pubic hairs is a personal choice. It is wise for us to experiment and see what works best, even if that means doing absolutely nothing at all. Prior to any procedure, thorough research is vital for helping us make informed decisions. Simply following our inner guidance leads us to enjoying a unique yoni-do!

Note: Electrolysis and depilatory creams are not recommended for yoni hair care. Electrolysis is very painful and takes a long time, whereas depilatory creams burn the hair off through a chemical reaction that can be very irritating to the skin.

Sperm's Role in Our Yoni Care

How does male ejaculate affect our yoni? Sperm and prostate fluid make up the male ejaculate and is **alkaline** in nature. This alkaline fluid can disrupt the **acidic** environment of our vagina and as our vagina works to re-acidify herself, there may be a temporary increase in smell. The more frequent and diverse the **sperm-baths** are (from multiple partners), the harder our vagina has to work to re-acidify herself. Why do we want an acidic vagina? The acidic nature of our vagina protects her from bacteria and other microbes. Thus, the acidic environment is important for the maintenance of our vibrant, healthy yoni.

Making love with my long-term partner would often result in frequent ejaculation, anywhere from one to five times per day, everyday. What I found was that the scent and taste of my yoni would change from light, sweet and fragrant to heavy, sour or brine-like. Whenever we would be apart for a while, my yoni would clean herself out and return to a fresh and sweet state. Now I prefer that my partner does not ejaculate inside my vagina, both for hygiene and for the sake of intimacy (when a man ejaculates, he loses his vital essence, and often this will shut him down in his emotional center). All my past partners who practiced ejaculation control were much more energized and loving after sex than those who ejaculated.

Questions: Does your yoni experience frequent doses of sperm? What is the smell of your yoni a few hours after ejaculatory sex?

Unless pregnancy is on our menu, male ejaculate can be best utilized as a sacred salve for anointing the rest of our body. Drinking it is also wonderful and a personal choice. There is no need to worry about the calorie myth as most debates on the matter state that semen is nutrient rich with only five to seven calories per teaspoon!

Exercise: Sacred anointing

This exercise is only for those of us who love male ejaculate and who want to experience it externally.

For this exercise, we first allow our partner to release his elixir (ejaculate) on our face or breasts and massage it into our skin. Then, over time, we let his elixir dry and tighten on our skin until it is like a facial. We then wash it off after a half hour or so.

*I would recommend encouraging, with love and respect, our male partner to learn some of the basic **healing love practices**. This will enable him to keep up with our growth and also help him to conserve his vital chi or essence.*

Safe Sex and Our Yoni

The use of condoms can also change the taste and scent of our yoni. It is best to fully pleasure our yoni prior to condom penetration so that the latex, lubricant or spermicide flavor does not interfere with the sweetness of our yoni's juices.

However, some of us use condoms even for oral sex and have learned to make the taste of latex sexy and fun.

Healing Imbalances

BREATHING YONI

Another factor that can play into the health of our yoni is letting her breathe. It is important for us to wear cotton or breathable underwear and perhaps even go some days or nights without wearing any. We can heal recurring bladder and yeast infections by changing our diet and by not wearing underwear, especially non-cotton underwear. There is a common belief that chi is lost when we go without wearing underwear. However, if we do the Jade Egg practices, our yoni will learn to seal herself, thus, preventing the loss of chi. As sensual women, we experiment to see what works for us and our yoni.

> Questions: Do you use condoms and if so, have you noticed a change in the smell and taste of your yoni? What are the results of sleeping without underwear?

SUN-KISSED YONI

Exposing our naked yoni to the sun is an ancient Taoist practice that allows our yoni to absorb the *yang* energy of the sun. Mantak Chia states, "the sun's energy is very healing and soothing to the genitals." Our inner yoni is a moist, dark place where (bacteria, yeast, and fungus) can grow. Sun exposure helps to nourish this area by allowing the yoni to gently air herself out while absorbing yang chi. This practice is similar to exposing a cut

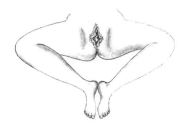

Fig. 11.2
Sunning the yoni

or an open area of flesh that is susceptible to infection to dry, clean, warm air. The morning sun is preferred because it is not as strong as the mid-day sun. If we enjoy nude beaches for extended periods of time, a little sunscreen on our yoni will protect her from a sun burn.

Exercise: Sun-bathing beauty

We can find a private place or a nude beach and open our yoni to drink in the pure yang force of the sun. But let's be careful not to overexpose our yoni and get a sun burn (see fig. 11.2).

Yoni Aromatherapy

Aromatherapy is an ancient art and science that uses pure plant essences to help our body return to a state of balance and vitality. Anointing or spraying our yoni with spritzes made from pure water and different aromatherapy can help our yoni maintain its radiant health. For example, a rose oil spritz sprayed on our yoni daily not only smells sweet, but is very healing and clearing for our yoni.

ESSENTIAL OIL USES FOR OUR YONI

Essential oils are pure plant extracts and most of them need to be diluted in water or a base oil before we apply them to our body. I have personally tested and used the following oils for my own yoni and her care:

Internal:
Lavender: clearing and healing
Tea tree: cleansing and healing

External:
Rose: loving and soothing
Sandalwood: sexy

Yoni Aromatherapy Recipes

INTERNAL USE

We can apply lavender and tea tree to a tampon for infections. It is important to dilute the oils as follows:

- ✧ Lavender: a couple of drops in a spritzer of pure water or in a few drops in some pure almond oil.

- ✧ Tea tree: a couple of drops in a spritzer of pure water or in a few drops in some pure almond oil.

EXTERNAL USE

We can spray the outside of our yoni and pubic hairs or apply a few drops directly on our hair (avoiding direct skin contact). Dilute as follows:

- ✧ Rose: just a couple of drops in a spritzer of pure water.

- ✧ Sandalwood: leave undiluted or mix with some pure almond oil.

We must be careful with vegetable and nut oils as it is common for them to go rancid. This can create an imbalance in our yoni. We need to experiment as some of us can handle anything in our yoni, while others cannot.

CAUTION: Essential oils destroy latex. *Do not use essential oils* **when using latex.**

There are also special blends of essential oils that address specific issues. Consulting a certified aromatherapist for a blend to suit our needs and concerns may be helpful.

> Question: Which aromatherapy treatments will you integrate into your daily yoni care?

Partner Chemistry and Our Yoni

Sometimes the pH of our partner's skin is not compatible with our own. We can tell by the reaction of our yoni to our partner. A change in pH is always indicated by a change in smell and taste—normally she begins to smell and taste unpleasant.

STORIES: *Chemistry is important*

After being with a lover that was not compatible, it took me five days to return to my normal smell and taste, even though we had used a condom. With another lover, one with whom I did not use a condom, I found his vajra (penis) would burn me on the inside. This experience has only happened with a couple of different men, but it was uncomfortable enough for me to realize that our genitals were not compatible.

A close friend of mine also had a chemistry mis-match with her husband. She would get recurring soreness and yeast infections. Her doctor finally told her that sometimes the chemistry of partners isn't compatible and discomfort and yeast infection can result.

Using our Jade Egg enables our yoni to become more resilient and strong, making us less susceptible to infections and soreness. Also developing our self-love and ability to track our emotional changes greatly empowers our understanding of our body's many messages. As we become intimately more acquainted with our body through the Art of Succulent Living and the Jade Goddess teachings, we as sensual women, will come to realize that all our pain, disease and imbalances are energy contractions that can be tracked to an emotional root. By choosing to honor our body and by delving deep into our inner mysteries, we can transform our contracted chi and unwind it to return to the fullness of who we truly are.

Old Goddess Recipes For Our Yoni Healing

The following are some great old goddess recipes that have been used for a very long time by women, long before pharmaceuticals were available. Using garlic, cucumber, apple cider vinegar, and yogurt for treating yoni imbalances and infections is still a common and effective treatment.

> Question: How can you use natural home remedies as a way to learn about your body and support its healing process?

Application of Old Goddess Remedies

GARLIC: FOR CLEARING YEAST

We may skin a clove and place it inside our vagina, changing it every few hours. We can use a needle and thread to attach a thin string to the clove for easy removal. We must *not* cut the clove as it may irritate the sensitive tissue of our vagina. Also, making sure to use our finger, we can scoop out all the cottage cheese like yeast in our vagina and up around our cervix. Adding garlic to our diet (either eaten raw or taking odorless capsules) will also give a boost to our immune system. Most yeast infections are due to a lower immune system function and can be remedied by boosting our immune system with healthy food, supplements, pure water, exercise and getting regular rest.

Note: Capryl capsules (taken internally) contain caprylic acid that kills yeast. Organic extra virgin cold pressed coconut oil (taken internally) also contains high levels of caprylic acid. This has been recommended as a quick and natural way to clear yeast. (for more information on capryl, look up Dragon's Den in the References)

Men are often carriers of yeast and bacteria. It is wise to treat our partner at the same time as we treat ourselves to stop the cycle.

CUCUMBER: FOR SOOTHING IRRITATION

Cleansing our yoni with a cucumber will also help restore her. This is great for mild irritations, as well as for supporting our yoni in her self-cleaning process.

To treat her with cucumber, we skin a cucumber and cut it into a slice the size of our pinky finger or smaller and clean all the seeds off of it. After inserting the cucumber into our vagina, we change it after an hour or so. We can also use a needle and thread to attach a thin string to the cucumber for easy removal.

APPLE CIDER VINEGAR: FOR RE-ESTABLISHING VAGINAL pH

Douching with apple cider vinegar can also help our vagina. However, we must not over do this as douching can also clear out healthy bacteria. If our vaginal wall is irritated, this douche can further irritate our vaginal lining. However, many women have successfully used an occasional douche to clean out their vagina when necessary. It is not necessary for us to do this frequently or on a long-term basis. Using our common sense and self-awareness will help us to determine the number of douches our yoni requires.

Dilute a tablespoon of organic apple cider vinegar with eight ounces or more of pure water. After the douche, insert a vaginal suppository of probiotics (found at health food stores).

YOGURT: FOR SOOTHING OUR INNER TISSUES

Organic, plain yogurt is extremely soothing to our inflamed and irritated yoni. It also contains healthy bacteria that will support our yoni to re-establish her healthy flora.

We can apply yogurt externally and/or internally, then rest on a towel, wiping off the yogurt after twenty minutes or longer. Taking oral or inserting vaginal probiotic suppositories can also help our body reestablish its healthy flora.

Helpful Tips For Prevention

The best medicine is preventative medicine. Making sure that our hands and our partner's hands are clean when touching our yoni will help to prevent the transference of germs into our yoni. For oral sex, making sure both partners also have clean mouths since sometimes our mouths and tongues can transfer germs to our yoni and our partner's vajra. Immediately after sex, it is a great practice to urinate (flushing out any germs that may have traveled up our urethra) and to wash both our own and our partner's genitals. The cleaner we are, the more we ensure a healthy yoni.

Practicing sex when we are emotionally imbalanced can also lead to infections. Yeast infections are often linked to anger and can sometimes be cleared by facing our anger and transforming it. Our emotional wellbeing plays a huge factor in the health of our genitals. By doing the six healing sounds combined with the sexual reflexology, we greatly empower our yoni to clean herself and return to her natural state of vibrant health. Any act of violence towards our yoni definitely lowers her immunity and creates a negative pattern that can embed itself quite deeply in her tissues. Touching our yoni when we feel positive and loving towards her empowers us as sensual women to participate in our yoni's healing.

Question: With what attitude do you touch your yoni?

Our G-spot: The Goddess or Sacred Spot

The G-spot, otherwise known as the Goddess spot or sacred spot, is connected to our urethral sponge. Through sharing the Jade Goddess teachings with many women around the globe, I have been able to observe a phenomenon with this sacred sponge in our yoni. What do sponges naturally do? Sponges absorb. The tissues of our sacred sponge/spot are especially susceptible to any negative sexual or emotional experience. Our sexual practice can provide us with a way to release old blockages and restore the vitality of our yoni. (for ambrosia anatomy, see Chapter 12).

It's Not All In Our Head

There is one very common female imbalance that I would like to highlight here that many women and medical professionals do not recognize as important. Here is a letter written to a women's sexual health center, "are you aware of a condition called vulvodynia? The symptoms are burning, pain and sometimes itching in the vulva, plus pain during intercourse or even on contact. To date, most common symptoms are vulvar dermatoses, cyclic vulvitis, vulvar vestibulitis (pain in the entrance to the vagina), vulvar papillomatosis and vulvodynia (or vulvar pain)." Basically, this is an irritation of our vaginal tissues that ranges from mild discomfort to extreme pain upon touching and especially with penetrating the yoni. Often, this is misdiagnosed, and we are sent to a sex therapist or psychologist to remedy our *problem*. If we suspect we may have this imbalance, we can mention it to our doctor.

Question: Do you experience physical pain with penetration?

STORY: Transforming our tissues

A woman had a severe case of vestibulitis. She could not tolerate any penetration and yearned to have a normal sex life. Through doing a lot of self-healing using the ability to move her own chi through her genitals, she was able to heal the raw nerve endings and enjoy a healthy sex life. If we suspect that we may have such an issue, we may want to research this material on-line by Googling volvodynia, vestibulitis, etc. There are many books and resources available to assist us in healing and empowering our bodies to become vibrantly healthy.

Caution and the Wisdom of Our Yoni

It is important to make sure we have the best understanding and care for our body. If we have an odor that is unpleasant, experience any pain or discomfort, or suspect any imbalance in our yoni, it would be wise for us to consult a health care professional. Most yoni imbalances are easily remedied if they are caught in the early stages.

There is an observable and direct relationship between illness and negative emotions and thoughts that are locked in the tissues of our body. Through this understanding and practice, we can clear cramps within minutes as well as painful irritation from yeast infections. If we can heal on the energetic level, we often find our physical body responds accordingly. Of course, we should also consult with a health care professional as to how to care for our body during an imbalance. It's important for us to understand what is happening to our bodies and to make wise choices on how to act to initiate the full healing of our body.

Menopause

Menopause to us modern women is often a dreaded time, and it is even often viewed as an unavoidable disease. Yet menopause is a natural and beautiful part of our feminine birthright. The worst aspect of modern menopause is how it is converted into yet another "female problem" that has become big business for the pharmaceutical companies. But therapies such as hormone replacement do not make sense. Do men have to take hormones to fix their testosterone levels? No. However, many men do. So why would we need estrogen?

There are many fallacies about menopause and some wonderful books written by women for women on the topic help to dispel these myths. Menopause is viewed in esoteric tradition as being a time when we become most powerful, most juicy, most wise and alive. It is an honorable time worthy of our celebration.

Our body is infinitely wise. As we shift into our power stage (there are three stages: the *child* stage, the *fertile/mother* stage, and the *power/crone* stage) our body knows perfectly what to do in order to maximize its own vitality and succulence. With menopause there is no monthly loss of eggs, and though our eggs may deteriorate a little, they still contain the powerful ovarian chi—a very favorable expression of the power stage. While younger women lose large amounts of vital life force through moon-time, a sensual woman entering her power stage of life enjoys the natural inward redirection of her life force and is able to live in a very high state of being.

Questions: Are you currently in your power stage? What are your beliefs about this time of your life?

Exercise: Power Stage

Let's imagine a new view on our power stage. As sensual woman who are in the power stage, we no longer can have babies. Therefore, we are free to be sexual without worrying about pregnancy. It is a time when we have seen enough to grow wise and compassionate. It is also a time when our inward flow of chi empowers us to glow with inner knowing and power. We cannot be deceived as easily, and we do not accept behaviors that are dishonoring, disrespectful and heartless. We can see through tall tales into the source of a person's true intentions. This is very powerful.

This power can seem frightening to those who hide behind false ideas. It is difficult to manipulate and control those of us who know our power as women. But this is a new time: a time when we women of all stages accept our power and our beauty. Each stage of life is beautiful and has unique gifts to offer us. As power stage women practicing the Art of Succulent Living, we have more leisure time—time for all those things we put off while pursuing an education, a career, motherhood, etc. The power stage is truly a time which is ripe for our power to blossom fully.

Question: How does this new description of menopause feel?

Dryness, Lack of Tone, and Low Libido

If we have a look at our lifestyles as women over the first forty years of our life, we can see that poor diet, poor exercise, poor self-esteem, lack of freedom to honestly express ourselves, and de-hydration all play a role in our sexual health and vitality. Through re-hydration, exercise, healthy food, and working with our inner energies through the Jade Goddess teachings, as sensual women we can find ourselves feeling younger and juicer. Being connected to sexual energy directly empowers our body to revitalize itself. Many sensual women have reported being wetter, more toned, and more interested in sexual energy after practicing with the Jade Egg. Even if having another lover may not be of interest or possible, it is still possible to circulate our sexual energy and become our own best lover.

Note: Kenalog in Orabase is a prescription ointment that some older women use to heal and lubricate their inner labia when they experience pain due to friction caused by walking. If a more natural solution is desired, aloe vera gel is also a great lubricant and healing salve.

> *Questions: How does it feel to know that we have the power to change our lives? What is the value in taking total responsibility for the results in your life?*

Our Breasts

Now that we have explored caring for our sexual centers, we are wise to explore our love center: our breasts. Our breasts are considered our love center because they sit on either side of our heart and represent the external expression of our heart chi. Chi naturally flows from our heart center out into the world. Our breasts have long been a symbol for nurturing and loving energy. They also hold the secret to our longevity.

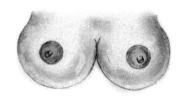

All of our breasts are beautiful—every shape, every size, every color is beautiful. Massaging and caring for our breasts regularly helps to harmonize our hormones, fill our breast tissue with chi, and open our heart. It also helps us to clear any stagnant chi in the tissues of our breasts and can prevent the formation of bumps, and thus, the prevention of breast cancer. Massaging our nipples activates our endocrine system and aids in the production of lubrication in our yoni. Furthermore, breast massage allows us to develop self-nurturing qualities, sending our loving attention inward instead of continuously sending it outwards to others.

I have been asked if our breasts—more specifically our nipples—are a source or opening from which we lose chi. Our nipples are actually a kind of sponge. What do sponges do? They absorb what they come in contact with. It is purely my own speculation that the rise in breast cancer is partially encouraged by the absorption abilities of our nipples drawing negative chi into our breasts. We live not only in a physically toxic environment (pollution, etc), but also a psychically toxic environment where negative emotions and thoughts are rampant. Just think of a situation where we are in a room and someone who is angry or depressed walks in: everyone can feel the energy of the room change. We seldom are aware of how much we dump our emotional/psychic toxins onto others. As women, we may naturally absorb these psychic toxins through our nipples. Therefore, breast massage with loving, smiling energy is important to the maintenance of our healthy tissue.

Of course, factors such as under-wire bras, anti-perspirants, diet, and our own mental and emotional state also influence the health of our breasts (and the rest of our body). In the Taoist viewpoint, the Taoists see that we are all part of the whole; this is also true for the body—all parts belong to the whole and affect each other.

Breast massage is not only vital for the physical health of our breasts, it also supports the maintenance of health for our whole body. Plus, it is fun! Some of my students have spent the first fifty years of their life only having their doctor or partner touch their breasts and have never explored their own body. We may be uncomfortable at first with touching our own breasts, yet with practice we find great lightness and joy in this experience. If this cannot be done for our pleasure, then let's do it for the maintenance of good health.

Questions: Have you been able to sense different qualities of energy in a person or place? How do you touch your breasts? What are the feelings you have when you do touch your breasts?

We penetrate the world with our breasts, whereas we receive the world with our yoni. Our breasts penetrate our partners, friends, family, and co-workers and open their hearts. It is vital for us to have a positive communion with these lovely mounds of love.

BREAST MASSAGE TECHNIQUES

The following is an in-depth description of the ancient secret practice of breast massage. Touching our breasts with loving attention and enjoyment is the core of the exercises and another tool for the sensual woman.

CAUTION: Women with any kind of breast lumps or cysts must ONLY massage in the in-up-outward direction. The out-down-inward direction is the expanding direction and may cause lumps and/or cysts to grow.

CULTIVATION OF HEART CHI AND HORMONES

Breast massage can be done seated or standing. If we are seated, we can roll a towel and place it so that it presses on our labia and clitoris as we sit. If we stand, we can begin by first massaging our clitoris and labia to generate a little aroused chi.

Warming our hands by rubbing them vigorously, we imagine them to be the ambassador of our heart, spreading love and warmth to our breasts. We massage using our Lao Gung (P-8) point in the palm of our hand. This palm point is more powerful then using our fingertips as it is connected to our heart/pericardium meridian.

Special note for women with mascectomies: It is very important for us to bring love into the remaining tissues and we can do this with a daily gentle massage. The use of rose oil combined with a soft inner smile to our heart will facilitate the flow of love chi into our cells and aid in renewing our sacred connection to our body.

SIMPLE VERSION

We massage our breasts in both directions, first circling from the inside out, then from the outside in (except if we have breast lumps or cysts).

TRADITIONAL TAOIST VERSION

We begin by circling outward and upward for 36-360 circles, and then reverse by first rubbing our hands again, then circling inward and downward 36-360 times. The first direction disperses energy, thus helping us to eliminate lumps and bumps and stagnant chi. The other direction is energizing and regulates our breast size (see CAUTION on page 207). Some women find their breasts getting larger, some firmer after doing this exercise.

While circling, we smile to our breasts and to our master glands in the center of our brain and allow our ovarian chi to move upward to these two places. During our breast massage we keep our tongue on the roof of our mouth while squeezing our yoni and anus. Inhale-squeeze, exhale-relax.

ELABORATE BREAST MASSAGE MEDITATION

PART ONE: NIPPLE (ENDOCRINE) MASSAGE

This elaborate breast massage and meditation is for maximizing our mastery of our hormones and sexual energy. We begin with part one by stimulating our hormonal system and by focusing on our nipples. We then follow this with part two, in which we connect with our organs through our breasts tissue.

Warming our hands while squeezing our perineum to awaken our sexual energy, we generate more mild aroused energy

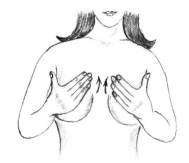

Fig. 11.3
Nipple/endocrine massage,
Lao gung on nipples

(mildly awakened ovarian chi) by massaging with our Lao Gung (palms) in circles over our ovaries until we feel them tingle. Beginning with our endocrine system, we barely touch our nipples with our Lao Gung/palms of our hands (see fig. 11.3 on page 208). Feeling the warmth of our heart chi (compassion) moving into our nipples, we massage in gentle circles moving inward, up, outward, down.

While circling over our nipples, we focus our attention on each of the different glands in our endocrine system (shown on fig. 11.4) and imagine each of our glands lighting up with chi:

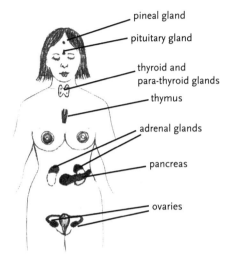

- ✧ crystal palace (master glands in the brain)
- ✧ thyroid/parathyroid glands
- ✧ thymus gland
- ✧ pancreas
- ✧ adrenals
- ✧ ovaries

Feeling all of our glands activated, alive and bright, we reverse the circles and

Fig. 11.4
Smiling to the endocrine system

imagine that we are inhaling up to our crystal palace and exhaling down to our ovaries. As we do this, we imagine that our sexual energy rises up through each of our glands as we inhale, and moves down through each of our glands as we exhale. Seeing (inwardly with our imagination) our chi moving as though our glands are all connected through one line of energy.

We smile as we are doing this, imagining all of our hormones balanced and youthful, then we rest for a moment.

PART TWO: BREAST TISSUE MASSAGE (ORGANS)

For part two, we continue massaging while moving onto our *breast tissue* itself, using the inward, up, outward, down circles. Our awareness moves into our heart and we feel the love and joy of our heart spread through our entire chest and breasts.

Using the creation cycle, we activate the virtues of each of our organs:

- ✧ Heart = love and joy
- ✧ Spleen = openness and fairness
- ✧ Lungs = courage and self-confidence

- ✧ Kidneys = gentleness and calmness
- ✧ Liver = kindness and generosity

Meditating and smiling the organ colors into our breast tissue:

- ✧ Red = heart
- ✧ Blue = kidneys
- ✧ Gold = spleen
- ✧ Green = liver
- ✧ White = lungs

We can also direct different qualities of our chi by altering the texture of our touch on our breasts:

- ✧ Warm loving touch with full palm = heart
- ✧ Firmly holding the breast tissue while circling shoulders = spleen
- ✧ Light finger tip touching, barely touching the skin = lungs
- ✧ Very gentle, kind and slow touching = kidneys
- ✧ Firm, vigorous circles = liver

Once all the virtues, colors and chi qualities are in our breasts, we reverse the circles and create the energy of compassion. We keep smiling, massaging and feeling compassion chi penetrate our tissue. Then we rest for a moment.

A Side Effect of Breast Massage: *Breast massage may lead to having firmer breasts. Enlargement is possible as well. The most potent fact is that breast chi becomes very powerful through cultivation, and those who have suckled them have reported feeling high for the rest of the day.*

SPECIALIZED MASSAGE STROKES

PSYCHIC CLEANSING AND LYMPH DRAINAGE

For this stroke, we visualize that we are clearing out any negative energy or toxins from the base of our breasts, through our nipples and out. We begin by holding the base of our breasts (against our body) and gently squeezing outwards to our nipples at least thirty-six times or more.

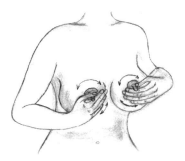

Fig. 11.5
Psychic cleansing and lymph drainage

PECTORAL TONING

Being aware of our pectoral muscles in our chest, we hold each breast gently, but firmly, making sure that our nipples are not covered. We press upward and diagonally inwards, then release gently while still holding our breasts. We do this at least thirty-six times or more.

This helps to tone our pectoral muscles which can give a lift to our breasts and also help clear more toxins or blocked chi in the muscle tissue behind our breasts.

UNCONDITIONAL LOVE

For this breast exercise, we gently hold each nipple while we imagine unconditional love flowing into our breasts (inhale) and out of our breasts (exhale). Breathing in deeply and slowly through our nose and smiling, we are aware of the energy coming in and moving out. It may feel like the chi is spiraling. We then rest for a moment.

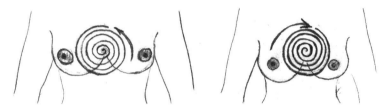

Fig. 11.6
Unconditional love spiraling in and out

FIGURE 8

Using one or both of our hands we trace a figure eight around both of our breasts with our heart being the center of the eight. We repeat the figure eight in both directions and then we rest for a moment.

AFTER MASSAGE TECHNIQUES

YONI POWER TO TRANSMUTE SEXUAL CHI

Resting and holding our breasts cupped in each hand we simply focus on breathing slowly in and out, squeezing our yoni and anus as we inhale, holding our breath and spiraling the chi in our master glands, and relaxing with our exhale. We keep sending our energy up into our breasts and brain, helping to transmute some of our sexual energy into compassion and rejuvenation. Dr. Stephen Chang suggests that "the exercise (breast massage with vaginal contractions) stimulates the production of the female hormone estrogen and causes it to spread throughout the vagina, uterus, breasts, and ovaries. One of the benefits is natural estrogen production. A surge in estrogen levels can greatly relieve the symptoms of menopause and rejuvenate a woman. The fact that estrogen is produced naturally is very important."

Possible Finishing Practice

We may choose to do our breast massage *prior* to our sexual foundation practices, specifically our ovarian breathing and ovarian compression exercises. These two practices combined with our breast massage enable us to further gather the rejuvenating chi of our ovaries. We can also do our breast massage without these two exercises and still get good results; however, for the best results, we must do all the exercises together.

Exploring and developing an intimate, nurturing relationship with our yoni and our breasts enhances our skills as a practitioner of the Jade Goddess teachings, as well as creates the space within us to deepen and expand our understanding of our own power and orgasmic potential as sensual women. As a last frontier of our journey together, we now turn our loving attention to exploring our sacred waters: our ambrosia or female ejaculate.

CHAPTER QUESTION

What was significant for you about the yoni (sexual center) care and the breast (love center) care?

CHAPTER TWELVE

Ambrosia

The Art of Female Ejaculation

Oh Goddess
your curves so full
your skin so silky beneath my touch
How can I feast upon you tonight?

I yearn to bite your tender flesh
and feel the essence of the Divine Feminine
seep onto my tongue
intoxicating me
head now spinning
delirious with delights
I crave more

May I caress the soft palace of ecstasy?
Placing my passion-flame within your mystery?

Igniting my soul, burning brightly
I sing a song once heard in ancient tongue
Goddess! Goddess!

How you fill me with precious drops of nectar, golden and potent
one drop alone is enough to send a shiver through the galaxy

stars don't twinkle it is their bliss you are witnessing
and I, oh I, yearn to be so lucky as they

To drink you in eon after eon
never full, never empty
always complete in your glorious beauty

AFTER GIVING LOVING ATTENTION to our breasts and our yoni, as well as deepening our continued practice of both the Jade Goddess teachings and the Art of Succulent Living, we are now ready to embark on the final frontier: discovering our sacred waters. Our ambrosia (female ejaculate) is still a subject of great controversy and research. Approaching this information with an open mind will give us greater potential to expand our understanding of the feminine mysteries.

How to Use This Portion of the Book

This final chapter is solely dedicated to the subject of our ambrosia, our sacred waters. The first portion of the chapter is devoted to the research and theory about ambrosia, while the second portion is devoted to the practice of activating our ambrosia. Reading through the chapter slowly and in its entirety is recommended before we attempt any of the practices given. Our attitude of openness, respect and curiosity will give us the advantage to explore this controversial subject with greater ease.

Ambrosia and Sacred Sexuality

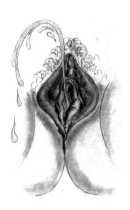

Before we begin broaching the theory and practical techniques of ambrosia, we must address an important issue concerning performance-oriented sex. The ancient art of ambrosia, now known as female ejaculation, has lost its sacred meaning through modern day exploitation in porn films and magazines. As sensual women making our way through the myriad of cultural beliefs on this subject, we come across a vast number of avenues that still objectify female sexuality. This chapter is a tool for transforming the objectification of the erotic feminine nature back into its sacred origins.

Questions: What has been your understanding of the subject of female ejaculation? Where did you get this information?

Another vital factor to address with the sacred art of ambrosia is a belief that all we women should ejaculate. It is important for us to understand that none of us need to express our ambrosia to feel fulfilled sexually. Thus, any person in the role of giving to us needs to examine their intentions as a giver and be comfortable with the fact that those of us who do ejaculate may not do so every time and that some of us never will. Rather than discussing the psychological reasons behind why our ambrosia will not flow, this chapter focuses more on the sacred act of sex and the mystery of the three sacred waters.

Questions: Do you ejaculate? If not, do you believe that you need to?

What is Ambrosia?

Authors Nik Douglas and Penny Slinger state, "woman has a limitless amount of Yin-essence, provided that she is in tune with nature." Ambrosia is an elixir produced naturally by our female body, and it is considered a sacred essence. To first understand our ambrosia, we must delve into the very nature of our female sexual essence. Our essence is yin in nature and resembles the ocean: deep, mysterious, watery. From having the power to host another life within us to accessing what seems like limitless bliss, our sexual power can seem frightening to those who don't understand it.

The ancient Taoists understood the nature of the feminine and describe it as being inexhaustible, cool, earthy, receptive and fertile. The concept of sacred erotic feminine essence has been lost to us modern women due to the imbalanced cultivation of primarily our yang, or more surface aspects of ourselves. Our lack of understanding is further enhanced by early social conditioning, sensationalized media messages, religious dogma and the limited education offered by Planned Parenthood in junior high.

Questions: Where and from whom did you receive your sexual education? Do you feel the messages given to you gave the impression that sexuality is sacred?

Most teens receive a basic education that covers simple sexual anatomy and some preconceived ideas about what sexual performance should look like. Traditional sex education is also filled mostly with horrific images of disease in order to scare the teens into being responsible. Unfortunately, due to this form of education combined with good girl/bad-girl upbringing and possibly religious dogma around self-pleasuring, most of us women end up devaluing our yin or softness and often feel that our bodies are inadequate. It is common for us to desire a washboard stomach, to try not to be so sensitive or emotional, and to be aggressive rather than loving in order to strive in the aggressive world. The "wham-bam-thank-you-ma'am" mentality of modern sexual habits has also played a part in keeping the mystery and sacredness of feminine sexuality and ambrosia undiscovered, or in some way hidden and repressed. What is still missing is our understanding of the deeper, subtler aspects of our sexuality. Although this holds little appeal to most, yin sexuality can actually lead to a much greater experience of erotic pleasure and to the activation of the three sacred waters (the three types of female ejaculate).

> *Questions: How do you feel about your softness and feminine curves? In what ways have you rejoiced in quiet, meditative sexual activity?*

Erotic Fingerprint

Our erotic fingerprint (our own sexual activation sequence or what "turns us on") is a unique expression of our sexual energy and is as diverse as our actual fingerprints. Knowing our own erotic fingerprint enables us as sensual women to clearly communicate our sexual needs and desires to our partner. Our tiny jewel of bliss (clitoris) is unique in its erotic fingerprint. Its location and sensitivity is at times mysterious for us women who do not know ourselves sexually and for our partners who are not aware of its importance. Our tiny jewel of bliss contains a unique secret code that is part of our erotic fingerprint. Unlocking her code is part of getting more familiar and comfortable with our sexual selves. Our ability to relax in sexual activity is largely due to our having a deeper understanding and acceptance of our own unique sexual responses. This dispels our fears of the unknown and allows us to receive more fully.

> *Questions: What is your erotic fingerprint (what turns you on)? Are you able to share this with your partner? What does the idea of sharing how you enjoy being pleasured feel like?*

Juicy Eroticism

Our relationship with our heart and our yoni is very powerful in enabling us to create more succulence in our sexual expressions. The more open our heart, the more juicy our yoni. This is true as well for the production of our ambrosia: the more love involved, the more ejaculate produced.

Why does opening our heart lead to our yoni producing more sacred water? We find the answer in the advanced alchemical Taoist practice of Kan and Li (water and fire). This practice blends our kidney (Kan/water) chi and our heart (Li/fire) chi to create a steam that induces orgasmic responses in our brain and body. The more open our heart, the more heat or fire there is to warm up our cool sexual waters (ruled by our kidneys). Whether or not we practice this advanced alchemy, the truth of how the open, warm essence of our heart activates our cool, sensual essence of our yoni remains as a workable guideline.

> *Questions: Have you noticed that when you feel loved and loving that your sexual experiences are heightened? Have you found this relationship of the heart and yoni creates more juiciness in you?*

Ambrosia: More Details Please!

Now that we understand that our ambrosia is natural and sacred, we can investigate its physiological and energetic source. The field of sexology has extensive speculation and debates on the topic of our ambrosia. Much research into this subject has revealed surprising results in attempt to explain what the Taoists call the three sacred waters.

The Three Sacred Waters

Both Taoist qi gong and Western medicine understand how the formation of the ovaries and testes occur in the kidney tissue and drop down with the development of the fetus. Recently it has been found that when the fetus differentiates into a male, a sponge-like tissue forms into his prostate and wraps itself around his urethra. In a female fetus the same tissue also wraps around her urethra, creating the urethral sponge (corpus spongiosum). Both the urethral sponge (female) and the prostate (male) have the same ducts within its tissue. Dr. Gary Shubach writes, "A number of researchers—in Israel and the USA—have established that tissue of the G-spot area contains an enzyme that is usually found only in the male prostatic glands. This may indicate that we are dealing here with a 'female version' of the prostatic glands, a collection of glands which also in men is rather sensitive to touch and pressure."

This first surprising result regarding our urethral sponge, as stated by Rebecca Chalker, finds that "female ejaculation comes from up to thirty or more tiny glands embedded in the urethral sponge, the tube of spongy erectile tissue that surrounds the urethra." The reason for this was explained in the development of the fetus. Just as massaging the men's G-spot (prostate) causes prostate fluid to be secreted, stimulation of the women's G-spot activates these tiny glands to secrete a fluid. Dr. Shubach confirms that "the G-spot in women is analogous to the prostate in men; like the prostate, the G-spot can produce a fluid-like semen (but not as viscous) which may be released on orgasm."

> Question: How does understanding that both men and women produce a prostate-like fluid upon having their "G-spot" stimulated help you understand your own physiology?

The second surprising result demonstrates that our kidneys are activated to release a non-urine substance into the bladder itself. This finding is documented by Dr. Shubach. He writes: "The clear inference was that the expelled fluid is an altered form of urine, meaning that there appears to be a process that goes on during sensual or sexual stimulation and excitement that effects the chemical composition of urine ... (causing it to) lose the appearance and smell of urine due to the secretion of the hormone aldosterone...." This result is an important link between Western medicine and Taoist understanding, in which our kidneys store our Jing (sexual) chi. Thus, our kidneys are responsible for creating sexual secretions.

> *Questions: Have you ever felt like peeing during sex? How does the information about the altered form of urine impact your understanding of your sexual fluids?*

As explained, Western medical research basically disagrees with the two possible locations of where ambrosia is believed to be created in our body—in our urethral sponge or in our bladder via our kidneys. Both of these findings are important in that they show that our ejaculate is indeed not urine. This contradiction is resolved when the Taoist understanding of our female sexual energy is applied to the research.

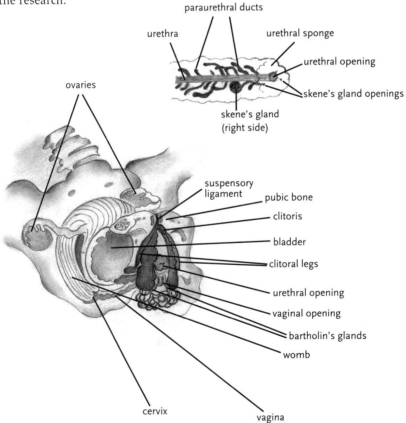

Fig. 12.1
Ambrosia system

A key Taoist concept is that the three sacred waters each have their own activation gate. The first water is depicted as coming from the stimulation of the first gate: our clitoris. This activates our para-urethral ducts which empty into our urethra and our skene's glands, glands that have their own openings on either side of the urethral opening.

Stimulation of our second gate, our G-spot or G-crest (located on the upper wall of our vagina) releases our second water. Often when this area is massaged, we have the sensation that our bladder is full. This makes sense as our kidney's are producing ambrosia through the release of the aldesterone hormone during arousal.

Our third water is connected to the stimulation of our third gate, our **epicenter**, which located on the front-top side of our cervix. Western research has not yet mapped this out, yet researchers speculate that our vaginal walls, cervix and uterus (all of which produce different discharges throughout our cycle) are the source of our third water. When our cervix and epicenter are stimulated, a very deep orgasm occurs and our third water is produced and released. However, Newman Kunti Lin, Ph.D as states, "female ejaculation from the vagina/uterus requires a powerful (level six or seven) orgasm, as we have experienced, to squeeze out the fluid stored in the porosities of the vaginal lining and uterine wall." Perhaps the fact that many of us women never get to this stage of arousal is in part why no Western research can be found on this third water that Taoists are so fond of.

Question: *How does the Taoist perspective on the three sacred waters help you to understand your female essences?*

Ambrosia as Sacred and Healing

Dr. Stephen Chang emphasizes that "according to Taoist teachings, every part of the body is holy." Unlike Western society's clinical perspective on sexuality, Taoists view sexual energy as an essential part of our daily life, a part that should be consciously cultivated for our health and vitality. We are seen as the expression of yin energy and our juices are pure yin essence. This yin essence is very healing to our body. As Dr. Stephen Chang further explains, "when the yin energy increases, negative ions are generated. Together these stimulate the parasympathetic nervous system, resulting in decreased blood pressure, slower heartbeat and breathing". Revering the power of our ambrosia as a perfect elixir for healing and harmonizing the body is part of the Taoist's perspective. For a person who has excessive yang energy, ingesting our ambrosia with its yin essence can serve to rebalance and harmonize them.

Western Medical Interpretation of What Taoists Call Healing Elixir

The healing elixir of which the Taoists speak is connected to the rejuvenating quality of alkaline substances. As Theodore A. Baroody, Ph.D, confirms, "The countless names of illnesses do not really matter. What does matter is that they all come from the same root cause...too much tissue acid waste in the body!" Examining ambrosia helps us to understand why the ancient Taoists considered it a healing elixir. Dr. Santamaría Cabello study on female ejaculate clarifies that "the fluid collected at the point of orgasm (distinct from the urine samples) showed the presence of PSA (prostate-specific antigen) in 100 per cent of samples", while Peter Faletra's shares on the composition of prostate fluid, "the prostate secretes a liquid that contains a number of enzymes, citric acid and calcium. This fluid is added to the semen during ejaculation and since it is alkaline..." These findings indicate that ambrosia is similar to prostate fluid and alkaline in nature. Taoists knew that most imbalances in the body were linked to over acidity. They also understood that ingesting an alkaline fluid that is rich with hormones (ambrosia) has harmonizing and rejuvenating effects on the body.

Question: How does understanding ambrosia as a healing, alkaline substance shift your perspective on female ejaculation?

Is Ejaculation for Every Woman?

Now that we better understand both the Western medical and Taoist viewpoints on ambrosia, we may feel greater acceptance of our sacred feminine essence. As sensual women, we must also honestly examine whether or not ejaculation is something we are personally attracted to. Some of us may doubt that we can even do it, whereas others may relax knowing it is indeed within our sexual potential to experience our ambrosia. We see this if we look at the physiology of our sexual anatomy. We all have the same parts: womb, ovaries, vaginal canal, labia, clitoris, urethral sponge, para-urethral glands, skene's gland, and so forth (unless they have been surgically removed). The actual physiological function of producing ambrosia is definitely within the capability of each of us; however, we may not all wish to experience this form of sexual expression.

For those of us who desire to experience ambrosia, but until now have been unable to do so, this may be due to the lack of development or activation in our sexual glands due to under-stimulation, infrequent use, or not experiencing higher levels of orgasms. Also, it is more common for some of us women to experience the release of our first and/or second waters (urethral ejaculation), whereas our third water (vaginal ejaculation) may not be as commonly experienced due to many factors. Newman Kunti Lin, Ph.D confirms the requirements for a third water orgasm: " the vaginal ejaculation requires a powerful PC muscle, a powerful multi-cycle orgasm, a high level of testosterone, and an optimal level of estrogen." Through specific practices of the Jade Goddess teachings, including the use of our Jade Egg, we can build our pelvic floor, strengthen our vagina, and influence our hormonal health, all of which are necessary for the creation and release of all three sacred waters. As sensual women, we understand that the phenomenon of ambrosia is a *being*/yin experience, not a *doing*/yang experience. Through the letting go of our goal to experience ambrosia, we take the first step into actualizing the flow of our sacred waters.

> Question: Since release of ambrosia is within every woman's potential and is purely optional, how do you feel about this for yourself?

Activating Our Ambrosia

PREPARATION

Before beginning to activate our ambrosia either alone or with our partner, it is important to shift our approach to our sexual play from goal-oriented to process-oriented, from fitting it into a short session during our busy schedule to setting aside some uninterrupted time. Normally the length of time we dedicate to our sexual encounters reflects the busyness of our modern life: short, intense and to the point. To arouse our ambrosia, we need more time. The art and joy of foreplay, kissing, licking, stroking, massaging, nibbling, touching, and activating our entire body, is essential to getting our sacred waters to rise and begin to flow. By paying special attention to our neck, nipples and inner thighs we can activate our sexual hormones. The longer our foreplay is extended, the more succulent we become. Taoists are very fond of foreplay and know that with prolonged stimulation, the three sacred waters start to be produced.

ALONE OR WITH A PARTNER

Through coaching both individual women and couples in the process of inducing their sacred waters to flow, it is important to state that although no ambrosia may come, a new kind of orgasm is experienced—yin orgasm that is much deeper in texture and tinged with emotional colors. With this in mind, we can rest assured that a new flavor of our sexual expression will birth itself.

> Questions: Are you and/or your partner attached to a particular result? What result and why?

Sacred ambrosia ceremony

We begin by first setting aside some uninterrupted time, making sure that our phone is off and the doors are locked (if we are in a situation where someone could walk in). Then we set up our environment to be comfortable and sensual, with ample towels beneath us or with the use of an **incontinence pad** to help keep our bed clean and dry. This helps us not to worry and allows us to release our ambrosia as much and as freely as we desire. If we are really worried about our bed, we can practice in a bathtub for our first session.

If we are alone, using our Jade Egg helps in the activation of our sexual chi; however, we may use any toy we enjoy. Whether alone or with a partner, we begin by touching our whole body in a sensual and appreciative manner, allowing our breath to be slow and full and breathing into all our parts as they are touched. Stimulation of our breasts and nipples will activate our hormones and the use of saliva on our nipples brings a lot of chi to them. If we are with our partner, we invite them to spend time sucking, licking and kissing our breasts.

After arousing our body to the point where our yoni feels ready to be pleasured, we continue to move slowly, using our breath to guide our movement. If we use our egg, we make sure it has a string attached to it. We then begin to gently massage and explore both our labia and clitoris. Our partner can also both manually and orally stimulate our clitoris and we may want to pull back our hood gently to expose our tiny jewel of bliss.

During this first activation, we become aware of our front channel, tailbone, and back channel. Using breathing techniques combined with our awareness circulates our sexual energy through our micro-cosmic orbit and assists us in redirecting some of our intense arousal energy away from our clitoris and up to our brain and the rest of our body. Taoists link our clitoris to our pineal gland. Thus, clitoral stimulation and redirecting our aroused chi further enhances our orgasmic experience.

Some of us may wonder why we would want to move the energy away from our genitals. This is not seen as a pleasure-diminishing technique, but rather as a pleasure-enhancing one because it spreads our orgasmic feeling throughout our body. This also leads us to opening our heart more and surrendering more fully to our pleasure.

The rhythm of this session is like a wave, arousing until we are near orgasm, then relaxing and letting our pleasurable sensations move through our body. We use the quiet moments to connect our heart with our yoni and to breathe slowly and deeply. Patience on behalf of our lover and ourselves is part of the adventure of activating our clitoral ambrosia which comes from our skenes glands (either side of our urethra), our para-urethral glands, and/or our bladder. This liquid is very clear and light. Our first water (and orgasm) further stimulates the glands in our endocrine system to become alert and activated. This fuller activation is part of our process in experiencing **higher orgasm** (instead of a short lived, genital orgasm).

After our first gate and first waters are activated, activating our second gate (G-spot) is much easier. Using firm, gentle and patient stimulation with loving intent enables our second gate to activate. It is common for us to feel the urge to urinate during this session so clearing our bladder beforehand may ease our mind. This urge is linked to our kidneys activating their production of our second water (aldosterone transformed urine) and filling our bladder.

The key to encouraging our second water to flow is relaxation. Massaging our G-spot (goddess spot) is deeply sacred and can induce feelings of vulnerability and even anger. Having awareness combined with a warm, loving heart can be deeply healing. The more open and soft our heart, the more we relax. Both partners may breathe more deeply and encourage sounds to come from deep within both our partner's and our own body. Activating our throat center (voice) also lends to opening this gate and helps to further activate our sexual center (genitals). Rather than a Hollywood-style screaming and moaning, our sounds are best naturally produced through surrendering to our pleasure.

Our second gate can take anywhere from a few seconds to a half hour to open so it is vital that both people be comfortable. The very fact that time can play an essential role in our ambrosia flowing could be why many of us have never experienced it, particularly if we did not invest enough time and dedication into our pleasure. As stimulation is increased and we deepen our acceptance to our pleasure, our sacred waters will start to flow, from as little as a teaspoon to fully soaking our mattress. The taste of this water will differ depending on our health—the healthier our body, the clearer and sweeter our taste. Again, the more open we are in our heart, the more ambrosia we will release.

The opening of our second gate allows our third gate (the cervix) to activate. To fully access our third gate, we require the use of skillful fingers, a vajra (penis), or a dildo. All around our cervix are many mini **erotogenic** spots (bliss-spots) with our major one being the epicenter in front of our cervix (see fig. 12.1, page 219). We open this third gate by gently, but firmly massaging around this entire area, using slow thrusts or spirals and making certain our cervix is never directly hit. The Taoist screwing techniques (tiny spiraling of the sacrum) are ideal for this and tend to bring us more awareness and chi than just regular thrusting.

Direct stimulation of our cervix can result in an intense opening of our heart and may cause us to feel of love and vulnerability. The more we allow ourselves to open deeper into our own mysterious ocean and trust ourselves to guide our partner to our full activation, the more likely our third gate will open. In response to our deep uterine orgasm (considered level six or seven orgasm by Taoists), our cervix may open and close or begin to suck as it contracts in orgasmic release. This is a very, very deep sensation that can be followed by the release of our third water.

Activation of all three gates and the release of our three sacred waters is a very powerful experience for all involved. The sequence given is only a guideline with which one hormone may stimulate another to be released in a chain reaction. This is why the Taoists recommend opening the first gate, then the second and the third gates. This sequence also helps us to open up to our innate ecstasy.

Whether we are alone or with our lover, we have the choice to stop at this point of releasing our ambrosia, breathing and resting to allow for our absorption of the healing nectar (ambrosia) into our bodies (taken in through drinking, licking and massaging). The absorption period may lead us into more lovemaking and continue the flow of our sacred waters in an expression of the inexhaustible yin. Making love from this space is incredibly sacred and quite different in its expression then regular intercourse, it is easier to access our *higher orgasms* in this state.

Whether our journey into the ancient art of ambrosia activation is a solo or dual experience, it is always precious and deeply healing. Once our gates have been activated, we can access our sacred waters whenever we desire. The more practice we have, the more we will be able to let our succulence fill us. As sensual women, we then are able to expand our erotic fingerprint or potential to beyond-sex experiences, to the point where a sunset, a taste, a fragrance could activate our juices to flow.

Questions: How does understanding how your sexual anatomy works to produce different types of ambrosia enhance awareness of your own body? Were you able to make love in this soft, opening, unrushed way? How did it feel to do this?

The Benefits and Challenges Connected with Ambrosia

From the Western perspective, the first and second waters or urethral ejaculates, can occur with or without orgasm. Forced ejaculation and urinary incontinence both have depleting effects on our energy. However, in Taoist sexology, orgasm is part of the release. Techniques are used to increase our levels of chi and, due to our cultivation practice, orgasm becomes part of our experience of releasing our three sacred waters. This increase of chi makes orgasmic energy available to us as well as enhances our sexual responses so we can experience a non-forced release of ambrosia. Non-forced, surrender/orgasmic ejaculation have energizing effects on our body. The benefits of experiencing multiple levels of orgasm are numerous. Dr. Winnifred Cutler's endocrinology research suggests that regular orgasm have healthy benefits such as higher levels of hormones, improving the health of the cardiovascular system, supporting bone density, increasing the functions of the brain, boosting the immune system and enhancing skin tone. The actual release of our ambrosia is not essential for us to receive all the benefits, yet when we do release, especially our third water, a very powerful sexual healing and spiritual connection is experienced.

Aside from non-orgasmic, forced ejaculation, Western doctors have claimed that some ejaculate can contain urine due to urinary incontinence. The release of urine is not actually bad in and of itself, but the psychological issues of peeing during sex (such as embarrassment, fear, anxiety) are numerous and widespread. To prevent or reverse incontinence, we can explore exercises, like the ones presented in this book, to increase the tone and strength of our pelvic floor muscles. Those of us who ejaculate regularly, however, do have strong pelvic floor muscles, so the theory of stress incontinence would not apply.

Another possible setback to the release of our ambrosia is the loss of potassium. Dr. Gary Shubach states, "… due to the secretion of the hormone aldosterone during sensual/sexual arousal, causing the re-absorption of sodium and the excretion of potassium by the kidneys." We can replenish our potassium by eating bananas or taking potassium supplements. If we experience exhaustion due to forcing our ambrosia, we can remedy this by making sure that we release our goal to ejaculate. We can cultivate energized ejaculation by our letting go, surrendering, and building the levels of orgasm in our body. Also of great importance is the concern of dehydration, which we rectify by staying fully hydrated and drinking plenty of water afterwards.

Questions: Do you feel tired after ejaculating? Are you too afraid of "peeing" to relax into experiencing your ejaculate?

The Importance of Sexual Energy Cultivation

Taoists have long recognized the potency of our sexual energy and the healing qualities of our sexual fluids. They also recognize that cultivating a positive attitude along with orgasm increases our vitality, libido and creativity. They view ambrosia as being a natural function of our awakened feminine essence that is not a goal for us, but a result of harmonized hormones, powerful pelvic muscles, and our acceptance of our fluids as natural expressions of our body. Simply understanding the true nature of our ambrosia will allow us to experience greater pleasure and relaxation during our sexual exchange.

Mantak Chia shares, "women have the capacity for virtually inexhaustible sexual pleasure, far greater than the capacity of men." As Western research increases our understanding of the physiological expressions of our female sexuality, Taoist sexology practices in turn enhance our hormones and increase the health of our sexual organs. A combination of both, along with the unique Jade Goddess practices, allows us as sensual women to tap into our inexhaustible (yin) sexual potential, regardless of our choice to release our sacred waters or not.

CHAPTER QUESTIONS

Is your new understanding of the physiology and esoteric properties of ambrosia helpful?

How does understanding that ejaculation is a choice and not a necessary part of female sexual expression effect your experimentation?

Do you feel confident that you can teach a partner about your sacred gates and the corresponding waters?

Come with me
Beneath the surface
Don't be afraid
Relax

Let yourself go
Open gently and feel me everywhere
I dance around you
Through vibrations of purest light
I enter you
We are one
We have always been one

Now that you remember
Let go
Open a little more
Feel yourself melt
Merging with all that is
To be everywhere and no where all at once

Letting go
Totally open
Feeling the subtle play of light upon your skin
There is only joy here
Pure, simple, beautiful

Now you are free
To go as you please
Just remember the song
The dance
The breath

Love is all there is
Joy is the pure expression of all that is

LOVE

Time and space collide and compress and in its midst,
Wholeness vibrates.
It is from this space our new journey begins.

We live in a time where the emergence of sensual women is greatly needed. When we choose to view our world through the philosophy of the Art of Succulent Living, we initiate the first step to healing the Feminine in all of us. This new paradigm invites us to explore how the world shapes us as women, and despite how things have been in the past, how we now can choose to express our feminine essence with integrity and power.

Once we awaken our desire to access our omni-orgasmic potential, our journey to cultivate our most precious resource, our vital life force (sexual chi), begins. Through our practical application of the Jade Goddess teachings, we enhance and harmonize our physical, mental, emotional, and spiritual selves and embrace all that it means to be a woman.

It has been said that in order to be instruments of great change in the world, we must first begin with ourselves. Many of us who believed we were helpless to change the conditions of our world now realize that it is through our own awakening that we can support the evolution of humanity. No greater task can be asked of us now. How wonderful it is that such a journey, rich with beauty, bliss, inner peace, and radiance, embodies our emergence as sensual women.

The following interviews are from four women who felt the desire to share their intimate experiences with other women for the purpose of inspiring and supporting the healing of the feminine.

Name: Linda
Occupation: Secretary/Student of the arts
Age range: 40s
Geographical location: Philadelphia

How did you come to practice the Jade Goddess teachings?
I did an internet search for goddesses and I found Saida's website. It was ideal timing because I had always been interested in studying a sexual-spiritual practice. Like the old saying, when the student is ready, the teacher will appear.

Was it what you expected? What happened as you practiced?
I did not know what to expect, but I was very happy with the results. I loved Saida's teaching style. She is warm and open and loving. I felt her loving presence from the moment I first met her, and she hugged me and said Aloha. As I practiced, I felt myself becoming more centered and calm. People would want to be near me (I was not used to this, and so it felt uncomfortable at times) or they would stare at me. I got used to the idea that they were responding to my new inner glow.

Did you have specific issues that were resolved through your practice?
I had not been sexual for many years and felt very closed down and sad. I felt myself opening up to this sexual energy in a way that I could handle. It wasn't an over the top, always horny type of sexual energy, but a gradual, more calming energy, something that I could handle. I did not have to worry about becoming uncomfortable or scared about working with or opening up to my sexual energy.

Do you consider this work valuable for women?
I think that this kind of work is extremely valuable for all women. Women have to learn to empower themselves sexually first. I grew up expecting that a man would provide me with a certain amount of love, sex and intimacy, and when they didn't, I would feel bad about myself. Having this kind of practice helps you to get in touch with your sexual energy and to work with it, so that you are empowered going into a relationship. You know that your needs will always be met, whether or not you are in a relationship.

Do you think this work would be for the everyday woman or only for those on a specific path?
I think that this would work for all women. Women need to understand their own bodies and their special energies. You do not need to have a certain belief or follow a spiritual doctrine to practice or benefit from these exercises.

What was the most important piece for you?
Learning to feel the energy, learning to become centered, learning to love and value myself.

Do you see yourself continuing to cultivate your sexual energy?
Sometimes as women, we can get so busy attending to everyone else that we forget to take time for ourselves. Having a support group would remind me to take the time to nurture myself and stick with my practice. When I am practicing, I enjoy it so much that I see myself as always having this as an important part of my life well into my golden years.

Has your sex life improved? The other aspects of your life?
I am not in a relationship now and that is by choice. Practicing has changed my life because I am not willing to settle for a relationship if my needs are not going to be met. In the past, I would have held on to a relationship just to have someone, and the kind of men I attracted were not giving. Now, I will not stay in a relationship if it doesn't feel right. My inner happiness has become more important.

What other significant pieces do you wish other women to know about?
I would tell other women to take the time to get to know themselves in a different way from what they are used to. They will come to know how special they are. Our sexual energy is a part of us and we should get to know this energy and be comfortable with it and to work with it for our benefit. When women are in touch with the positive aspects of themselves everyone benefits.

Name: Heather R. Dawn
Occupation: Ecstatic Movement & Relationship Coach
Age range: 30s
Geographical location: Los Angeles

How did you come to practice the Jade Goddess teachings?
I went to the Divine Feminine Teacher Training where Saida taught me the Jade Egg practice.

What happened as you practiced?

I found that my sexual drive started to increase slowly and my wetness increased. The great thing that happened with using the Jade Egg is that I was able to separate my vaginal muscles and notice that I could squeeze either all or one set of muscles and this was very helpful in love making and self pleasuring.

Did you have specific issues that were resolved through your practice?
I wanted to have more vaginal wetness and a stronger sex drive and the wetness did improve. So I'm grateful for these things improving in my life. Plus, I did want to strengthen my vaginal walls, and it has definitely helped me with that.

Do you consider this work valuable for women?
Yes, most definitely. For many reasons, not just what I've mentioned above, but to be more in touch with their yoni and their sex. To empower themselves more in many ways: sexual, acceptance of their bodies, and being more in charge of how their body works so that it is a more blissful place.

Do you think this work would be for the everyday woman or only for those on a specific path?
I feel that every woman could benefit from this work on some level, even if it's just body acceptance and awareness of their yonis. I think every woman could benefit somehow from this work, as it's the place most people avoid, even in massage. There is much healing to be done in this area of most women's bodies.

How did your partner respond to your changes?
He loves them! Better sensations, stronger, and it's great to give him a massage from the inside.

What was the most important piece for you?
Increased wetness and the strength of my vagina walls and seeing that I can separate my muscles and squeeze different areas—top, middle and bottom, or all of them together. It's fun!

Do you see yourself continuing to cultivate your sexual energy?
Oh, yes, yes!

What other significant pieces do you wish other women to know about?
Just to have patience with the process, as it does work. It just may take some time. Having more patience heals much with the body and the heart. I feel the Jade Egg mixed with the Taoist practices are very calming, loving and energizing to the soul, body and mind all at the same time. There is so much healing to be done, so much letting go in this work. It's about being present, patient and loving with oneself. The push only causes more pain, and it's time to let go of the pain and let go into the pleasure and healing.

Name: Anna Thea
Occupation: Teacher
Age range: ageless, Born 1960
Geographical location: Las Vegas

How did you come to practice the Jade Goddess system?
I took the Divine-Feminine certification program where Saida introduced us to the Jade Egg practices.

Was it what you expected?
I didn't really know much about it and had no expectations.

What happened as you practiced?
It has changed my life and my attitude about my Sexuality! It helped me to release old patterns of shame that were literally stored in my yoni. In the process I taught myself how to ejaculate. I have a much more intimate relationship with my yoni and the egg has definitely deepened my sexual response.

Did you have specific issues that were resolved through your practice?
I developed a healthier, sacred, and more loving attitude about my yoni.

Do you consider this work valuable for women?
This work is very important for all women. It brings light (a crystal egg) where there is darkness and consciousness where there is all to often confusion, misinformation, and shame. This work is extremely valuable!

Do you think this work would be for the everyday woman or only for those on a specific path?
I believe every woman should incorporate some form of this practice. It is about learning to love ourselves more deeply, literally at the "root" of our being.

How did your partner respond to your changes?
Over the time that I have been practicing with the egg I have not had a sexual partner. I feel that the egg has played an instrumental role in expanding my sexual consciousness and in attracting a more sexually conscious mate into my life and with those that I have engaged in outercourse with they have often commented on the tone and strength of my yoni.

What was the most important piece for you?
The egg has completely changed my relationship with my yoni. I have a much more intimate and loving relationship with my body and my yoni and a level of consciousness and mastery over my sexual energy and female anatomy that I never knew possible. I love having a healthy, responsive, toned yoni. I can feel more deeply different parts of my yoni and my sexual energy is much more

expanded. I now use the egg without needing a string and I treat my egg as a sacred friend.

Do you see yourself continuing to cultivate your sexual energy?
Yes. I believe it will be a life long journey of exploration.

Has your sex life improved?
Most definitely! These practices have provided me with profound sexual healing and have really tuned me in to what my yoni needs in order to respond.

The other aspects of your life?
I see how my sexual energy is intertwined in all that I do. How I express my sexual energy is how I manifest into the world. If my sexual energy is heart centered, sacred, and celebrated then my whole life is too.

What other significant pieces do you wish other women to know about?
Honoring our yoni and having a sacred relationship with her is the most precious gift we can give ourselves and our beloved. Knowing what our yoni needs and really honoring her and giving her a safe place to express herself is crucial. As we do this, the men in our lives will benefit immensely and have the greatest honor, devotion, and respect for us.

Name: N.T.
Occupation: Acupuncturist
Age range: 30s
Geographical location: Los Angeles

How did you come to practice the Jade Goddess teachings?
I was introduced to the system by Saida during a retreat. I had done qi gong for years and had heard of Taoist sexual techniques, but I did not think they were accessible to a non-yogi/Taoist like myself. I am an average modern chic.

Was it what you expected? What happened as you practiced?
I didn't have any expectations when I started the program. I do know the general benefits of qi gong to the body's energy system, but I had never done any work specifically on the reproductive system.

Did you have specific issues that were resolved through your practice?
I experience a level of fear and insecurity about not achieving orgasm. After a few sessions using the practices of the Jade Goddess, and in only the first thirty to forty minutes of work, I noticed I was more grounded, and I was able to let some of that angst go for that moment and just enjoy my lover.

Do you consider this work valuable for women?
Most definitely. As a practitioner of acupuncture and herbs, I see many women with physical manifestations of emotional trauma from abuse and just living who report irregular menses, painful menstruations, fibroids, and who are either not sexually active or not in touch with their sexuality. Prior to practicing and learning of Saida's work, I knew that this was a lower jiao stagnation or holding pattern that is treatable with acupuncture, herbs, and qi gong. It is my opinion that this practice is a valuable adjunct to any medical program designed to strengthen and tonify a woman's reproductive health, which is linked to her sexual health.

Do you think this work would be for the everyday woman or only for those on a specific path?
I think that women who are searching for this type of work will benefit from this practice as part of their path and will find it sooner. However, I think that all women share a similar path in that we all strive for love and beauty in our lives. Aren't we all just everyday women?

How did your partner respond to your changes?
My partner and I have been intimately involved for over two years, so we are very in sync with each other's sexual response. My partner was very aware that I was experiencing something a little different, because he was also! The first pattern that was different was that I experienced an orgasm that was not the typical explosive very contractive orgasm I usually experience with him, but instead it was a more subtle implosive "tease" orgasm. It was the sensation of orgasm without the strong vaginal contractions. Because I figured he didn't feel it and I was exited, I was quick to share my experience. He said that he did feel my vagina contract, but not as strong. The second noticeable experience was two nights ago when he was giving me oral pleasure (yeah! :)) and he had his fingers inside my vagina. After I climaxed, he said that while he was fingering me, "I totally opened up" for him. He said that sometimes when his fingers are inside of me it feels like he hits a wall, but at one point, my whole vagina just opened up for him. He was very excited to be so graciously invited! Aside from the sexual benefits, I enjoy the exercises because, like all qi gong practice, I can get quiet and focus on my body and my emotions. I am learning to be more centered while pulling chi into my ovaries and vagina instead of just releasing stagnant chi.

What was the most important piece for you?
I am already receiving the benefits and I haven't even started to use the egg. I am doing the exercises sans egg. My body isn't ready for that yet. I really like the energy clearing with the color and sounds. It is just like clearing energy from the yin organs. I am aware that my emotions get stuck in my pelvis at times and I must clear them out.

Do you see yourself continuing to cultivate your sexual energy?
Most definitely. I look forward to taking a class with Saida.

Has your sex life improved?
Yes.

What other significant pieces do you wish other women to know about?
That the sexual benefits are only one part. Qi gong is a complete system and clearing from the vagina and pulling chi through the body benefits all aspects of health. And really, I want women everywhere to know that health problems are physiological AND emotional. Qi gong is an invaluable tool for emotional energy transformation. The path is not the path of a yogi or a monk. It is the path of learning to be human.

Here are some tips for juicy daily living. We can use the ones that inspire us the most as a daily meditation.

Juicy Tip #1:   Love yourself no matter what.

Juicy Tip #2:   Let go of needing a reason to be joyous, and express your natural joy.

Juicy Tip #3:   Delight in every moment, every person, and every experience.

Juicy Tip #4:   Remember to smile: circulate and radiate your vital life essence.

Juicy Tip #5:   Be the love and acceptance you seek.

Juicy Tip #6:   Wear your egg and rejuvenate yourself in every moment.

Juicy Tip #7:   Keep your tongue on the roof of your mouth as often as possible.

Juicy Tip #8:   If imbalanced emotionally, do the healing sounds until balanced.

Juicy Tip #9:   Breathe deeply and allow your orgasm to permeate all of you.

Juicy Tip #10:   Nature is in a constant state of ecstatic aliveness. Join in.

Juicy Tip #11:   Massage your breasts every day, spreading love to every cell.

Juicy Tip #12:   Your body is your sacred temple; your choices are your worship.

Juicy Tip #13:   Express your unique beauty every day, in all things you do.

LIST OF PROFESSIONALS AND EDUCATION CENTERS

Taoist Education

Mantak Chia and Universal Tao Instructors, Universal Tao Center
www.universal-tao.com

Michael Winn and Healing Tao Instructors
www.healingtaousa.com
www.HealingTaoRetreats.com

Rachel Abrams, M.D.
www.multiorgasmicwoman.com

Taoist Health

Healing Tao Center, Herbs for Sexual Health
www.taohealing.com

Dragon's Den, Supplements for Healing Yeast
(1) (808) 572 2424 (world-wide shipping)

Tantra and Transpersonal Psychology

Divine Feminine Institute, Caroline Muir and Joan Heartfield, Ph.D
www.divine-feminine.com

Transforming Beliefs

Option Institute, Barry Neil Koffman
www.option.org

Women's Empowerment

Judith Ansara Gass MSW, founder of Sacred Union, empowerment training and
retreats for women and couples
www.sacredunion.com

Dr. Christiane Northrup, author of *Women's Bodies, Women's Wisdom*
www.drnorthrup.com

Patricia Taylor, author of *Expanded Orgasm*
www.expanded-orgasm.com

A-frame orgasm An orgasm where the top of the vagina pushes down and out; normally associated with female ejaculation.

Acidic The pH balance of less than 7.

Ajna The point between the eyebrows (mid-eyebrow point).

Alkaline The pH balance of more than 7.

Aroused practice Jade Egg practice while feeling sexually aroused or excited.

Bai Hui (Bah-Hoo-way) The crown point, or point found at the top of the head when the chin is tucked in; sometimes a point where energy is held and spiraled to energize the brain.

BDSM (Bondage S&M) Bondage sado-masochism; the use of bondage in dominant and submissive play to achieve altered states of bliss.

Bio-feedback A connection between the body and the mind that uses an external part of the body in order to distinguish what is happening internally.

Bone marrow nei gong (Nay-gong) A cultivation practice that uses internal energy to enhance bone marrow, blood and energy.

Bulbocavernosus muscle A superficial perineum muscle that contributes to opening and closing the vagina and to creating orgasmic sensations.

C-7 The 7th cervical vertebrae in the spine; an energy-refining station in the micro-cosmic orbit.

Cauldron An energy collection point, located two or three inches below the navel and deep inside the belly, where the pearl (condensed chi) is stored.

Cervix The mouth of the uterus.

Chi (chee) Simply means energy.

Clitoral system The system of nerves in the genitals and pelvic floor that is connected to the clitoris.

Clitoris glans The tip of the clitoris.

Coitus The physical union of male and female sexual organs that leads to orgasm and the ejaculation of semen.

Creation cycle The cycle of chi flow wherein the organs support and enhance each other; the cycle flows from the lungs to the kidneys to the liver to the heart to the spleen, then this pattern repeats itself.

Crystal palace The master glands in the brain which include the pineal, pituitary, thalamus, and hypothalamus.

Cum-passion A play on the words cum (orgasm) and passion (love) meaning the alchemy of sexual energy and love creates compassion energy.

Dead zones Areas of the psyche and body that are locked into habit patterns.

Divine God or Goddess, the concept of wholeness and of the sacred.

Divine Feminine Goddess, feminine principle of God, the sacred feminine.

Divine Masculine   God, masculine principle of God, the sacred masculine.

Dominant   When a person initiates sexually and enjoys leading.

Dual cultivation   The exchange of energy during sexual union with a partner.

Ego   The lower emotions, the unaware self, the feelings of superiority.

Energetic cords   Unseen energy connections between people; this can be supportive as in the love of a mother with a child or can be destructive as in the exploitation of another for bettering oneself; unseen energy can be cleared through qi gong practice and other energetic techniques.

Energizer breathing   Quick breathing that heats up the body.

Epicenter   Anatomical point near the cervix, located on anterior (front) wall of vagina.

Erotogenic   Areas that are erotically sensitive.

Essence   The core of who we are, the animating spirit within us.

Etheric   The electro-magnetic field that corresponds to the atoms of physical matter, also known as the energy body. A common example is feeling pain in a 'ghost' body part (a missing limb).

Formula   A specific practice developed by Taoists known to yield specific results.

Fountain of Youth   The practice of rejuvenating and revitalizing the body so that it can regenerate and heal itself and thus appear younger; an internal fountain of youth is found in the energy contained in the eggs which are contained in the ovaries.

G-crest   Coined by Dr. Gary Shubach, the G-crest is the entire urethral sponge, an area that encompasses the entire anterior (front) portion of the vaginal canal; this area can be activated to be sensitive and pleasurable.

G-spot   The Grafenberg or Goddess spot found in the vagina; this spot causes intense sexual pleasure when stimulated.

Healing love practices   The sexual qi gong practices found in the Universal Tao system, for men and women, recommended here for men who wish to learn more about ejaculation control.

Higher orgasm   Orgasms beyond the level of pelvic contractions; subtle and refined orgasms that may or may not include genital and muscular response.

Horse stance   A martial art posture that involves placing the feet wider than hip-width or shoulder-width apart and bending the knees, while keeping the back straight.

Hui Yin (Hoo-way-Yin)   The perineum point, or the point found between the vaginal opening and the anus, also referred to as the Gate of Life and Death; when it is open, it is believed that energy is lost (death); when it is sealed, it is believed that energy is contained within the body (life).

IUD   An intrauterine device used for birth control.

Imperial fire   The fire energy from the heart center; not a literal fire.

Incontinence pad   A pad used in hospital and care homes for those with incontinence; one side is soft cotton, the other side, either rubber or plastic, making the pad liquid proof.

Jade Egg   An egg-shaped piece of natural Jade.

Jing chi (Ching chee)   There are two forms of Jing chi (energy) Prenatal Jing is the original energy created when the sperm and egg meet and unite to create life, and acquired Jing is the energy created through eating, sleeping, exercising and positive life experiences.

Kan and Li (Kahn and lee)   This refers to water (kan) and fire (li) and the ancient practice of inner alchemy wherein the water and fire energies are brought together to create a healing steam (energetic not literal water, fire or steam).

Kundalini syndrome (Koon-dah-leen-ee)   When the dormant life force (kundalini) awakens without proper preparation and/or circulation, it can cause the nervous system and brain to 'short circuit' and lead to imbalances ranging from the physical, psychological, emotional, and spiritual.

Lao gung point (Lahow gung)   A point found near the center of the palm, connected to the pericardium meridian (therefore, linked to the heart energy).

Life-enhancing   Anything that adds to vitality, energy, and life.

Life-giving   Anything that creates more vitality, energy, and life.

Life-taking   Anything that depletes vitality, energy, and life.

Love vibration   The energy of our heart that we define as the feeling of love.

Lust-full   The opposite of feeling lust (our own energy); desire to be filled by another's lust.

Master glands   The pineal, pituitary, thalamus, and hypothalamus glands in the brain, which are the master glands that direct the rest of the systems of the body.

Micro-cosmic orbit   The circuit of energy that runs from the perineum up the spine to the brain and back down the mid-line of the front of the body back to the perineum.

Meng mein   The point along the micro-cosmic orbit that lies directly across from the navel, on the spine, just below the kidneys.

Natural   Free from pretension or artificiality: spontaneous.

Orgasm   The peak of sexual stimulation; the experience of intense energy rushing through the body; the feeling of relaxation and profound aliveness.

Outer labia   The outer lips of a woman's genitals.

Ovarian palace   An energetic collection point in the center of the uterus/womb.

Oxytocin   A hormone released by the pituitary gland when women spend time together (also released during breast feeding) that causes feelings of being nurtured; is a hormone that promotes bonding.

Palpating   To touch with the desire to sense or feel the tissue.

PMS   Premenstrual syndrome which includes symptoms such as irritability, breast soreness, and bloating; any symptoms of discomfort prior to menstruation.

Pure   Free from contamination and foreign elements.

Qi gong (chee gong)   Energy practice; an ancient Chinese practice of cultivating different energy and of refining and circulating these energies within the body for better health, balance and vitality.

Sex chakra (sha-crah)   The energy center located at the genitals.

Sexual bonding   The connection formed during sexual union.

Slaying the Red Dragon   The ancient Taoist practice of eliminating menstruation, and now refers to the elimination of PMS symptoms.

Sperm-baths   When sperm is applied externally to any part of the body.

Solar plexus   The soft area just below the sternum, where the rib cage ends.

Stagnant chi   Any energy that is blocked or stuck in our body.

Source   The creative Universal force from which all life originates.

Submissive   When a person enjoys receiving and being guided sexually.

Succulent   Juicy; full of vitality; exciting; energetic.

T-11   The 11th thoracic vertebrae in the spine; an energy-refining station and pump in the micro-cosmic orbit.

Tan tien (Dahn tea-en)   Elixir field; an energy point at the navel where energy can be directed and collected; in this book, we refer to the lower tan tien located below the rib cage down through to the pelvic floor.

Taoist (Dow-ist)   People of Chinese descent who lived according to the wisdom of nature; scientists and artists who developed longevity and vitality through cultivating their energy.

Taoist sexual qi gong (Dow-ist chee-gong)   The ancient practice of cultivating sexual energy for longevity, vitality and spiritual evolution.

Throat chakra (sha-crah)   The energy center located in the throat, at the thyroid and parathyroid glands.

Thrusting channels   Energy channels that run up the left and right sides of the body (internally) starting at the perineum and exiting at either side of the Bai Hui point or crown point on the cranium.

Un-aroused practice   Jade Egg or sexual foundation practice that is performed while feeling un-aroused sexually and that involves accessing ovarian energy without sexual excitement.

Urinary incontinence   Losing urine when laughing, sneezing, and making love due to weak pelvic floor muscles.

Uterus   The womb; part of a woman's genitals where a fetus grows into a baby.

Vajra (Vah-je-rah)   Sanskrit word for penis; refers to the male principle.

Yabyum (Yab like Cab-Yum)   A Tantric posture involving a woman sitting on top of a man with her legs wrapped around his hips; an ideal position for meditating and circulating energy.

Yang The masculine principle in Chinese medicine: hot, active, male.

Yin The feminine principle in Chinese medicine: cold, still, female.

Yoni (Yo-Nee) Sanskrit word for the female genitals, sacred temple.

Abrams, Rachel Carlton M.D. and Mantak Chia. *The Multi–Orgasmic Woman*. Emmaus, Pennsylvania: Rodale Press, 2005.

Avinasha, Bodhi and Sunyata Saraswati. *Jewel in the Lotus, The Tantric Path to Higher Consciousness*. Fairfield, Iowa: SunStar Publishing Ltd, 1987.

Baroody, Theodore A. N.D., D.C., Ph.D. *Alkalize or Die*. Waynesville, North Carolina: Holographic Health Press, 2002.

Chalker, Rebecca. *The Clitoral Truth*. New York, New York: Seven Stories Press, 2000.

Chang, Dr. Stephen T. *The Great Tao*. San Francisco, California: Tao Publishing, 1985.

Chang, Dr. Stephen T. *The Tao of Sexology, The Book of Infinite Wisdom*. San Francisco, California: Tao Publishing, 1986.

Chia, Mantak and Maneewan Chia. *Awaken Healing Light of the Tao*. Huntington, New York: Healing Tao Books, 1993.

Chia, Mantak and Maneewan Chia. *Healing Love through the Tao, Cultivating Female Sexual Energy*. Chiang Mai, Thailand: IHT Publications, 1986.

Cutler, Dr.Winnifred. Athena Institute, Chester Springs, PA, July 2006. http://www.athenainstitute.com/discoveries.html http://www.eroticuniversity.com/healthorgasm.html (accessed July 2006)

Dawkins, Richard. *The Selfish Gene*. New York, New York: Oxford University Press, 1976.

Douglas, Nik and Penny Slinger. *Sexual Secrets, The Alchemy of Ecstasy*. Rochester, Vermont: Inner Traditions International, 1979.

DVA. "You and Your Prostate, Function of the Prostate Gland." Australian Government Department of Veterans' Affairs, 2001. http://www.dva.gov.au/media/publicat/2001/prostate/ch1.htm (accessed July 2006)

Élysa enr. "Consultation, A Condition called "Vulvodynia." Department of Sexology at the Université du Québec. http://www.unites.uqam.ca/dsexo/english/9811e/qa0224-0206m.htm (accessed July 2006)

Faletra, Peter. "Male and Female." Department of Energy United States of America. http://www.newton.dep.anl.gov/askasci/zoo00/zoo00061.htm (accessed July 2006)

House, Random. *Unabridged Dictionary*. New York, New York: Random House, 1993, Inc.

Jarrett, Lonny S. *Nourishing Destiny*. Stockbridge, Massachusetts: Spirit Path Press, 1998.

Kaplan, Hilary. "Tampons, an unpublicized health hazard." Yale Daily News Publishing Company, April 9, 1999. Yale University. http://www.yaledailynews.com/article.asp?AID=1366 (accessed July 2006)

Kaufman, Barry Neil. *To Love Is To Be Happy With*. New York: Ballantine Publishing Group, 1977.

King, Francis. Tantra for Westerners, *A Practical Guide to the Way of Action*. New York, New York: Destiny Books, 1986.

Klein, Dr Laura Cousino and researcher Shelley Taylor. "Women & Friendship." Oregon State University. http://studenthealth.oregonstate.edu/news/womenandfriendship.php (accessed July 2006)

Ladas, Alice Kahn, Beverly Whipple, and John D. Perry. *The G-spot and Other Discoveries about Human Sexuality*. New York, New York: Dell Publishing, 1982.

Lee, Bruce. Wing Chun, Jun Fan, Jeet Kune Do, JF/JKD. http://www.wingchun.com/JKD.html (accessed July 2006)

Lin, Newman Kunti, Ph.D., PE. "Female Ejaculation." Lin Institute. http://www.actionlove.com/extra/ejaculate.htm (accessed July 2006)

Oleson, Terry, PhD, and William S. Flocco. "Randomized Controlled Study of Premenstrual Symptoms Treated with Ear, Hand, and Foot Reflexology." *Obstetrics and Gynecology*, Vol. 82, #6, December 1993. American Academy of Reflexology. http://www.americanacademyofreflexology.com/PublishedResearch.html (accessed July 2006)

Pacholyk, Andrew, MS, L.Ac. "Crystal Dictionary of Metaphysical Meanings, Jade." http://www.peacefulmind.com/stones.htm#J (accessed July 2006)

Physicians, Board Certified. "Definition of Orgasm." *Webster's New World™ Medical Dictionary*, First and Second Editions, January, 2003. John Wiley & Sons, Inc. http://www.medterms.com/script/main/art.asp?articlekey=11783 (accessed July 2006)

Piquemal, M., M.D., prepared by Christine Issel, "Global Effect of Reflexology on Blood Flow Research Study." *ICR Newsletter*, Vol. 15, No. 1, March 2006, page 18-19. http://www.reflexology-usa.org/articles/Piquemal_Article.pdf (accessed July 2006)

Santamaria, Dr. F. Cabello. 2001. "Female Ejaculation: Research Contrary to BBFC Ruling." Quoted in Louise Achille and Catherine Wilkinson, *Feminists Against Censorship*. http://www.fiawol.demon.co.uk/FAC/femejac.htm (accessed July 2006)

Schubach, Dr. G. Ed.D, A.C.S. "The G-'Spot' Controversy, The G-'Crest' and Female Ejaculation, The Experiment." 1997. http://www.doctorg.com/gspotcontroversy.htm http://doctorg.com/female-woman-orgasm/female-g-spot-experiment-5.htm (accessed July 2006)

Singer, J., and I. Singer. "Types of Female Orgasm." In J. LoPiccolo and L. LoPiccolo, eds., *Handbook of Sex Therapy*. New York, New York: Plenum Press, 1978. http://www.wordiq.com/definition/Orgasm (accessed July 2006)

Webster's 2. *New Riverside University Dictionary*. Boston, Massachusetts: Riverside Publishing Co., 1984.

Further Acknowledgments

The author gratefully acknowledges the assistance of Marina Fomchenko for her fabulous illustrations.

For more information about Marina Fomchenko, Illustrator:
http://www.tantricmoment.com

For comments and assistance, the author would like to thank Tannia Hecht.

For more information about Tannia Hecht, MA, *Pubic Hair Care*, Esthetic Educator: http://www.cara-mia.net

Jade Goddess
PRODUCTS

The Jade Egg

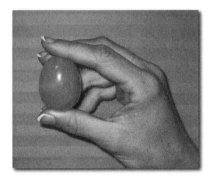

These beautiful, solid jade eggs, hand-carved and drilled to Saida's specifications, are the perfect tool for enhancing sexuality. Jade is known as the health, wealth and longevity stone renowned for protecting the wearer from negative energy. Previously only used by royalty in Ancient China, these precious eggs are now available to unlock the mysteries of your sexual chi.

Item JGJE01 $40.00 USD

Jade Egg Practice CD

This CD is a one hour, guided practice (Saida's voice) in which you are taken through a warm-up, lying down, seated, standing and completion practices. Many women have said that it is very easy to understand and follow. Highly recommended for women as a support tool for their continued practice and cultivation of their sexual chi.

Item JGCD01 $20.00 USD

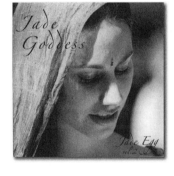

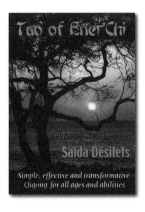

Tao of Ener'Chi DVD

This innovative DVD features 1.5 hours of instruction as well as 5, 10, and 15 minutes of daily practice routines. Designed for all ages and levels of experience, this is an exceptional tool in developing a personal experience of qi gong. Join Saida in beautiful, tropical Maui, Hawaii, and begin your journey of cultivating radiant aliveness today.

Item JGDV01 $25.00 USD

ORDER ONLINE AT:
www.jadegoddess.com

School Needs Identification Form

Name _____

☐ 11 Self Help Skills

☐ Don/doff coat or jacket

☐ Care of possessions

☐ Carrying books/supplies

☐ Independence in cafeteria

☐ Independence in bladder management

☐ Other (please specify) _____

_____

_____

Description _____

_____

_____

☐ 12 Social Acceptance

☐ Disability awareness

☐ Social skills training

☐ Overcoming social isolation

☐ Positive inclusion

☐ Social competence goals for IEP

☐ Hygiene

☐ Other (please specify) _____

_____

Description _____

_____

_____

School Needs Identification Form   Name _____

page 7

☐ 13 Social and Emotional Issues

☐ Adult dependency

☐ Medical noncompliance

☐ Self esteem

☐ Body self image

☐ Learned helplessness

☐ Manipulation

☐ Identifying genuine disabilities

☐ Socialization

☐ Blocks to independent functioning

☐ Work personality

☐ Organizational skills

☐ Promoting positive traits

☐ Other (please specify) _____

_____

_____

Description _____

_____

_____

☐ 14 Parent and School Relationships

☐ Home-school intervention

☐ Adjustment at school entry

☐ Enhancing communication

☐ Parent and teacher partnership

☐ Creating successes

☐ Other (please specify) _____

_____

_____

Description _____

_____

_____

School Needs Identification Form

Name _____

15 Transition Services

☐ Vocational assessment   ☐ Post high school training

☐ Vocational planning   ☐ OVR referral

☐ Transitional preparation   ☐ Other (please specify) _____

☐ Transitional planning

Description _____

_____

16 Other Needs

Please specify _____

Description _____

_____

_____

Comments

School Needs Action Form

The School Needs Action Form selects specific problems from the School Needs Identification Form and refers each problem to a particular specialist. It also provides for documentation of follow-up, including the plan, outcome, and date of closure.

School Needs
Action Form

Name of student _____ Date of interview _____

Name of interviewer _____

Problem(s) identified _____

Referred to _____
                    name

Area of specialization _____

Description of Problem
_____
_____
_____
_____
_____

Plan
_____
_____
_____
_____
_____
_____

Outcome
_____
_____
_____
_____

Date Closure
_____
_____

School Needs Progress Report

The School Needs Progress Report is basically a blank page for charting all of the work done with a given student, in chronological order. Each of the specialists addressing all of the problems designated on the action forms enters notes on these progress report pages.

School Needs
Progress Report

For internal use only

Student's name _____ Date _____

Area _____ Recorded by _____

Action(s) Progress Report _____

School Needs Outreach Program Visit Form

The School Needs Outreach Program Visit Form provides for the logging of home or school visits. One copy is included in the student's chart, and another is centrally filed to record all of the outreach work done.

S chool Needs
Outreach Program

Name ——————————————— Date of visit —————

☐ Home visit   ☐ School Visit

Reason for visit ————————————————————————

Staff member(s) involved ————————————————————

Summary of findings

Recommendations/plan of action

School Needs Release Form

The School Needs Release Form provides for prompt access to necessary information. It should be obtained from the parents as early as possible in the service delivery process.

Spina Bifida Association of Western Pennsylvania
320 E. North Avenue
7th Floor, South Tower
Pittsburgh, PA 15212
(412) 321-4900

School Needs
Release Form

Authorization for release educational records information to:
The Spina Bifida Association of Western Pennsylvania

I hereby authorize _____
print name of school

_____
Street   *City*   *State*   *Zip*
to release school record information to the Spina Bifida Association of Western Pennsylvania.

This information is to include records of _____ 's education or
name
treatment for the following time periods:

_____
Date

_____
Date

Check portions of records which are necessary

☐ Summary
☐ Educational-psychological
☐ I.E.P.
☐ Other_____

———— *Please Print* ————

Student's name _____

Student's address _____

Student's birthdate _____

Signature of parent/guardian _____

Witness _____

Unit/department _____

Date _____

———— *This authorization is effective for sixty days from the authorization date* ————

427

School Needs Team Staffing

The School Needs Team Staffing form is used to announce which students will be presented at team staffing.

$$S_{chool\ Needs}$$
Team Staffing

Date ———————————————

Place ———————————————

Time ———————————————

School Needs Summary
of School Staffings

With the School Needs Summary of School Staffings form shown on the next page, each student being served is assigned to one staff member who will be responsible for coordinating information and services. This assignment is based on the student's primary area of need. Any member of the clinic or association team may be assigned as case manager of a given student. This form identifies the caseworker, problem, and plan, and is used by the School Needs program coordinator to keep track of assignments.

School Needs
Summary of School Staffings

Name _____ Caseworker _____

Problem

Plan

Name _____ Caseworker _____

Problem

Plan

Name _____ Caseworker _____

Problem

Plan

Name _____ Caseworker _____

Problem

Plan

School Needs
Case Load Management

The School Needs Case Load Management form on the next page assists the program coordinator in managing the caseload by distinguishing between those cases that require only monitoring, those that are active, and those that are to be served on a priority basis. It also provides for supervision of the program coordinator.

School Needs
Case Load Management

Service Priority

Name	Case worker	Staffing date

Active

Name	Case worker	Staffing date

Monitor
quarterly/biannually

Name	Clinic date	Comment

Service Completed

Name	Date

New Referrals

Name	Ref date	Staffing date

School Needs Service Record

The School Needs Service Record form on the next pages is a monthly log of services delivered. It provides for oversight of operations and keeps records available for reporting to the board of directors, funding sources, and other bodies to which the association is accountable.

Spina Bifida Association of Western Pennsylvania
Spina Bifida Center of Allegheny General Hospital

Month _____
Name _____

School Needs Service Record

Date	Type of service	Type of problem	School/agency served	Family/child served	Location	Video Used?	Number in attendance	Staff providing service	Prep. time	Travel time	Test. time	Meet. time	Agency vehicle	Personal vehicle	Lodging	Meals	Tolls	Total	Comments

Service Identification Codes

NI	Needs identification	RK	Record keeping
IS	In-service training	PHC	Pre-hearing conference
CC	Case conference	DPC	Due process conference
IEP	Individualized education program	SV	School Visit
MDT	Multidisciplinary team meeting	TST	Testing
Ped	Parent group education	HV	Home visit
Ced	Community group education	Obs	Observation
INC	Information/consultation	CD	Curriculum development
SD	Staff development	L	Legislation
TSS	Team school staffing	OT	Other
CON	Case contact (telephone calls)	PC	Parent conference

Problem Identification Codes

1	Health related services	11	Self-help skills
2	Physical management	12	Social acceptance
3	Accessibility	13	Social & emotional issues
4	Safety & fire drills	14	Parents & school relationships
5	Preparation for school entry	15	Transitional services
6	Education, rights & related services	16	Other needs
7	Academic difficulties	17	Information and education
8	Pschological Assessment	18	Placement
9	Perceptual motor deficits	19	Language disabilities
10	Visual perception deficits	20	Transportation

Spina Bifida Association of Western Pennsylvania
Spina Bifida Center of Allegheny General Hospital

Month _____
Name _____

School Needs
Service Record

Date	Type of service	Type of problem	School/agency served	Family/child served	Location	Video Used?	Number in attendance	Staff providing service	Prep. time	Travel time	Test. time	Meet. time	Agency vehicle	Personal vehicle	Lodging	Meals	Tolls	Total	Comments

Materials Resource List

Culatta, B. *Guidelines for identifying language deficits in children with spina bifida.*(Adams Hall University of Rhode Island, Kingston, RI 02881)

How to Participate Effectively in the IEP Process (n.d.). Pittsburgh: Learning Disabilities of America.

Lord, J., Varzos, N., Behrman, B., Wicks, J., & Wicks, D. (1990). Implications of mainstream classrooms for adolescents with spina bifida. *Development Medicine and Child Neurology, 32,* 20–29.

McLone, D.G. (1986). *An introduction to spina bifida—McLone* (Spina Bifida Association of America, 1700 Rockville Pike, Suite 540, Rockville, MD 20852)

The most important meeting you will ever attend. (Western Instructional Support Center, 5347 William Flynn Highway, Gibsonia, PA 15044)

Special Education Check up—National Committee for Citizens in Education

Stauffer, D.T. (1984). Catheterization—a health procedure schools must be prepared to provide. *Journal of The Association for Persons with Severe Handicaps, 54*(1), 37–38.

Williamson, G.G. (Ed.). (1987). *Children with spina bifida: Early intervention and preschool programming.* Baltimore: Paul H. Brookes Publishing Co.

Index

Abstract (*verb*), 141
Abstract concept, 141
Abstract concept development,
  125–141
  comprehension of explanations
    and, 129–130
  deficits in
    assessment of, 130–134
    remediation of, 134–139
  experiential limitations and, 129
  factors influencing, 126–130
  perceptual deficit and, 126–129
  training in
    effectiveness of, 139–140
    exaggeration of defining charac-
      teristic in, 135–136, 137
    explanations of word meaning in,
      136, 138
    number of examples in, 135
    provision of reasons to notice
      examples in, 138
    real-world examples in, 139
    types of examples in, 136
Abstraction, perceptual, 184
Academic skills
  abstract concept development,
    125–141
  see also Abstract concept
    development
  language, *see* Language skills
  mathematic, 145–166
  see also Mathematic skills
  perceptual-motor skills and, *see*
    Perceptual-motor skills
  poor, low normal intelligence and,
    117–118
  progress in, social progress and,
    232
  success in, social acceptance
    affecting, 249
  see also Learning *entries*
Acceptance, social
  disability awareness and, 245–272
  see also Friendships; Peer interac-
    tions; Social acceptance
Access
  building, *see* Buildings, accessible
  to peers, 248

see also Social acceptance
  to school, 31–66
  see also School access
  to technology, elementary school
    programs and, 367
Accommodation, in parent–teacher
    partnership, 297
Action plan, 412
Active agent, 240–241
Active listening
  defined, 240–241
  in parent–teacher partnership,
    294–296
Active rehearsal, in problem-solving
    modeling, 164
Active status, 412
Activity(ies)
  adaptive equipment enabling, *see*
    Adaptive equipment
  alike-and-different, *see* Alike-and-
    different activities
  decubiti and, 20–21
  extracurricular, high school and,
    370
  fine motor skills and, 195, 196–197
  growth effects on, in adolescents,
    19–20
  organizational skills and, 205,
    224–225
  positive inclusion in
    in senior high school, 266
    in seventh and eighth grades,
      261–262
  unavailability of, social isolation
    and, 246
  visual-motor skills and, 198
  see also specific activities
Ad analysis, in disability awareness
    programs, 266–267
Adaptability, 319
Adaptation, of work spaces, 314–315
Adaptive coping mechanism, 241
Adaptive equipment, 31
  defined, 66
  designing rooms for accommoda-
    tion of, in disability awareness
    program, 258
  IEP and, 336